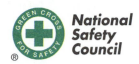 

Wilderness First Aid

EMERGENCY CARE
FOR REMOTE LOCATIONS

HOWARD D. BACKER, M.D.
Past President, Wilderness Medical Society
Department of Emergency Medicine
Kaiser Permanente Medical Group
Hayward, California

WARREN D. BOWMAN, M.D.
Past President, Wilderness Medical Society
Medical Director, National Ski Patrol
Cooke City, Montana

BRUCE C. PATON, M.D.
Past President, Wilderness Medical Society
Clinical Professor of Surgery
University of Colorado Health Sciences Center
Denver, Colorado

PETER STEELE, M.D.
Klondyke Medical Clinic
Whitehorse, Yukon Territory, Canada

ALTON THYGERSON, Ed.D.
Consultant/Medical Writer
National Safety Council
Professor of Health Science
Brigham Young University
Provo, Utah

Jones and Bartlett Publishers
Sudbury, Massachusetts
Boston • London • Singapore

Editorial, Sales, and Customer Service Offices

Jones and Bartlett Publishers
40 Tall Pine Drive
Sudbury, MA 01776
978-443-5000
Internet: http://www.jbpub.com/nsc/, email: nsc@jbpub.com

Jones and Bartlett Publishers International
Barb House, Barb Mews
London W6 7PA, UK

The first aid and CPR procedures in this book are based on the most current recommendations of responsible medical sources. The Wilderness Medical Society, The National Safety Council and the publisher, however, make no guarantee as to, and assume no responsibility for the correctness, sufficiency or completeness of such information or recommendations. Other or additional safety measures may be required under particular circumstances.

Library of Congress Cataloging-in-Publication Data
Wilderness First Aid: Emergency Care for Remote Locations/
Bruce C. Paton [et al].
      p. cm.
      At head of title: National Safety Council. Wilderness Medical Society.
      Includes index.
      ISBN 0-7637-0407-5
      1. Mountaineering injuries. 2. Outdoor life— Accidents and injuries.
      3. First aid in illness and injury.
     I. Bruce C. Paton. II. National Safety Council. III. Wilderness Medical Society.
RC88.9.M6W53 1998
616.02 ' 52—dc21   97-31077
                                          CIP

Emergency Care Editor: Tracy Murphy
Project Editor: Candace A. Kooyoomjian
Editorial Assistant: Karen McClure
Senior Production Editor: Cynthia Knowles Maciel
Assistant Production Editor: Rebecca S. Marks
Manufacturing Buyer: Jenna Sturgis
Marketing Director: Tara Woodman
Cover and Text Design: Nieshoff Design
Editorial Production Service: Books By Design, Inc.
Illustrations: Rolin Graphics
Typesetting and Pre-press: Pre-Press Company, Inc.
Front Cover Photograph: Mark E. Gibson
Back Cover Photograph: Bruce C. Paton
Printing and Binding: World Color Book Services
Cover Printing: Coral Graphic Services, Inc.
Additional Photo and Illustration Credits on page 332.

ISBN 0-7637-0722-8 (National Safety Council)
ISBN 0-7637-0407-5 (Trade/Jones and Bartlett)

Printed in the United States of America
01 00 99 98 97   10 9 8 7 6 5 4 3 2 1

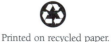

Printed on recycled paper.

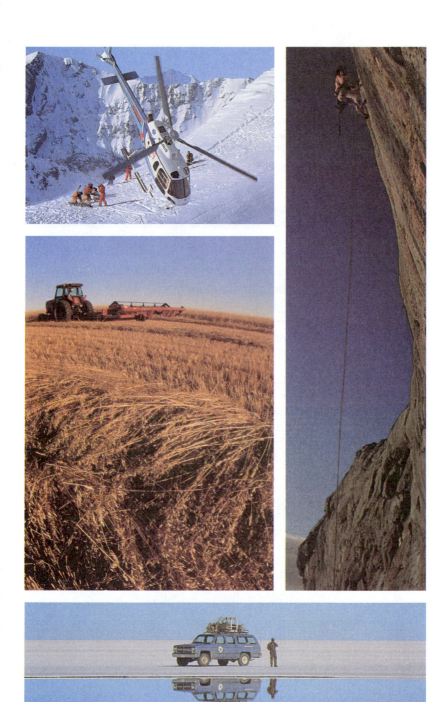

Contents

Bandaging the Wrist and Hand • Bandaging the Ankle and Foot • Applying a Dressing over a Wound without Pressure • Signs That a Bandage Is Too Tight

Contents continued

Acknowledgments

This text would not have been complete without the assistance of colleagues who reviewed and contributed to the manuscript:

Contributors

Gerard Glancy, M.D.
The Children's Hospital
Denver, CO

Robyn Goodfellow, M.D.
Department of Obstetrics
and Gynecology, Kaiser
Permanente Medical Group,
Hayward, CA

Luanne Hallagan, M.D.
Yellowstone Park Medical Service
Assistant Professor of
Emergency Medicine
George Washington University,
Washington, DC

Eric Johnson, M.D.
Emergency Medicine
of Idaho, Inc.
Boise, ID

Kevin Kogut, M.D.
Department of Anesthesiology
University of Washington
Seattle, WA

Joseph Serra, M.D.
Stockton Orthopedic
Medical Group
Stockton, CA

Eric Weiss, M.D.
Stanford University
Medical Center
Stanford, CA

James Wilkerson, M.D.
Merced Pathology
Medical Group, Inc.
Merced, CA

Reviewers

David Bates
Boy Scouts of America –
National Office, Irving, TX

Burt Hood
Arizona Chapter, National Safety
Council, Phoenix, AZ

Laura Kitzmiller
Texas A&M, College Station, TX

Steve Lyons
Wilderness Professional Training
Crested Butte, CO

Tom Myers
Grand Canyon National Park
Grand Canyon, AZ

Robb Rehberg
Advisory Board Chairman
National Safety Council
Ramsey, NJ

Steven Sarles
Chief Rangers Office
Yellowstone National Park
Yellowstone, WY

Donna Siegfried
First Aid Institute Manager
National Safety Council, Itasca, IL

Laura Slane
YMCA of the USA, Chicago, IL

David Webb
REI, Denver, CO

Holly Weber
SOLO, Wilderness Emergency
Medicine, Conway, NH

Carl Weil
Wilderness Medical Outfitters
Elizabeth, CO

Preface

Mike and Mary are hiking in Yellowstone National Park, ten miles from the nearest road, when Mike trips, pitches forward down a hill, and cuts his forehead badly. His face is covered with blood, but all Mary has in her pack are a handkerchief, one adhesive strip, and a water bottle."

People who travel, work, recreate, or live in the wilderness and other remote areas must expect that, sooner or later, they will have to deal with an injury or medical problem. **Wilderness First Aid: Emergency First Aid for Remote Locations** provides comprehensive information about how to deal with medical emergencies when help is hours — even days — away.

This book is a must for outdoor recreationists (hikers, skiers, hunters, climbers, rafters, fishers), for people who work in remote places (farmers, foresters, linesmen, ranchers), for people who live in areas (small communities, ranches, and vacation homes) where the EMS system may not be able to respond immediately to an emergency, and for travelers in countries where medical care may be inadequate or difficult to reach.

"Steve, a public service linesman, is working with his helper, Joe, along a remote dirt road 30 miles from town. Steve suddenly falls from the utility pole and lands on the ground, unresponsive. Luckily their truck is equipped with a radio, but Joe is faced with the terrifying dilemma of how to deal with Steve's injuries before help arrives."

This is not a wilderness survival book, although much of the information would help you survive if you were stranded unexpectedly. The information in **Wilderness First Aid: Emergency First Aid for Remote Locations** will provide you with the "what to look for's" and the "what to do's" needed to cope successfully with injury and illness.

The wilderness, national parks, and other remote areas of the United States are receiving more and more pressure from a population intent on using the "great outdoors" for fun, adventure, and travel. Rock climbing, river rafting, kayaking, and fly fishing are a few of the activities drawing millions into the wilderness. Unfortunately, many of these people are poorly prepared to deal with emergencies. Don't be one of the unprepared. Learn how to deal with emergencies before they happen.

Knowledge and understanding can prevent many accidents.

Preface continued

Much of the information in this book is different from what you might read in an urban first aid manual. Wilderness first aiders must be prepared to treat problems that they would not be asked to deal with when an ambulance is only minutes away. Some of the procedures are tagged as "Advanced." You need to know about them, but don't use them without additional training.

"Bill G. lives on a ranch. One day, while putting a horse into the corral, the horse lashes out with a kick that breaks Bill's leg below the knee. Hearing his cries for help, his wife, Emily, comes running out of the house. As she rushes to help her husband, Emily becomes panicked. The nearest help is two hours away and it's getting dark. What should she do?"

Prepare yourself for wilderness emergencies by taking a National Safety Council Wilderness First Aid course taught by a qualified instructor. Such a course varies in length, depending on how advanced you want your training to be. But, when the time comes, the time and money you spend could be one of the best investments of your life.

Introduction to Wilderness First Aid

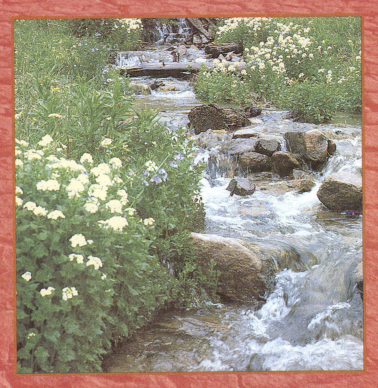

What Is Wilderness? • What Is Wilderness First Aid? • Legal
and Ethical Issues • Psychological and Emotional Issues •
Infectious Disease Precautions • Immunizations

What Is Wilderness?

Wilderness first aid is needed for activities in remote areas (hiking, climbing, camping, sailing, hunting, birding, snowmobiling). Anyone living, working, traveling, or just enjoying the wilderness should be prepared to manage a medical emergency. Broadly defined, wilderness is a remote geographical location more than one hour from definitive medical care. Such locations include remote areas where outdoor occupations are conducted (farming, ranching, mining, commercial fishing, forestry); remote communities; developing countries; and urban areas after a disaster destroys infrastructure and overwhelms emergency medical services (EMS).

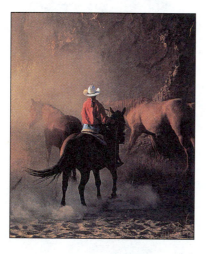

What Is Wilderness First Aid?

Wilderness first aid is the immediate care given to an injured or suddenly ill person. It does not take the place of definitive medical care. It consists only of giving assistance until a more advanced level of medical care, if needed, is obtained or until the chance for recovery without medical care is apparent.

Wilderness first aid has a distinct focus because

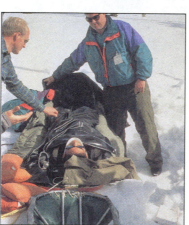

- injuries and illnesses occur outdoors, often in adverse conditions (heat, cold, altitude, rain, snow), that affect both victims and rescuers;

- definitive medical care may be delayed for hours or days by a difficult location, bad weather, and lack of transportation or communication;

- certain injuries and illnesses are more common in remote areas (altitude illness, frostbite, wild animal attacks);

- medical care beyond urban first aid may be needed (reduction of some dislocations, wound management);
- first aid supplies and equipment are limited;
- difficult decisions must be made (e.g., start cardiopulmonary resuscitation [CPR]? evacuate the victim?).

Most first aid books and training courses are designed for those with rapid access to EMS. In these cases, first aiders usually help for a few minutes, until an ambulance arrives; then their job is finished. However, wilderness first aid may require extended skills, depending on time, distance, and availability of medical care. A wilderness first aider may have to remain many hours or days with a sick or injured person.

Examples of Simple Measures That Can Prevent Serious Medical Problems

- Travel with a companion and let others know where you are going and when you expect to return.
- Do not use drugs or alcohol in the wilderness.
- Carry adequate food and water.
- Carry extra clothing and always anticipate a change in the weather.
- Learn route finding and avalanche avoidance for winter travel.
- Limit your rate of ascent at altitude and know the symptoms of altitude illness.
- Always ventilate a stove inside a tent or snow cave.
- Never approach or provoke wild animals.

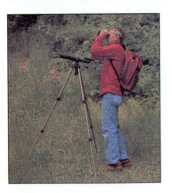

First aid involves treating not only others, but also yourself. Skillful first aid may make the difference between life and death, rapid recovery and long hospitalization, or temporary disability and permanent injury. Most important, wilderness first aid stresses prevention. Prevention will be stressed throughout this text, because it is much easier to avoid a problem than to manage an existing one.

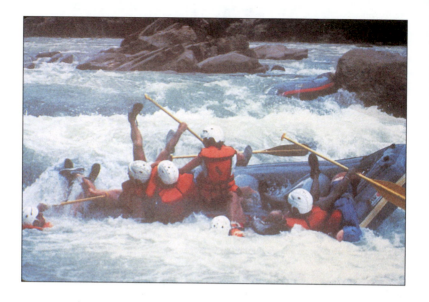

You must also learn that, unfortunately, you cannot treat or save everyone. Tragic accidents do occur, especially with high-risk wilderness activities. Nature is beautiful, powerful, impersonal, and can overwhelm and destroy as easily as thrill the wilderness traveler. The risk of death increases in a remote area with no access to advanced medical care, and some injuries or illnesses are fatal despite first aid efforts or rapid access to a hospital.

The information in this book will help you manage many common, minor problems and recognize more serious ones. A few advanced first aid measures are mentioned to allow some intervention in a desperate situation. Interested students, especially those responsible for others in the wilderness, are encouraged to continue their training beyond this text.

Legal and Ethical Issues

Fear of a lawsuit makes some people wary of helping in an emergency. The following legal principles govern emergency care.

1. You are under no legal obligation to aid a stranger. The decision to help in an emergency is usually a moral one.

2. A contractual or legal obligation—a "duty to act"—applies to park rangers, law enforcement officers, firefighters, and emergency

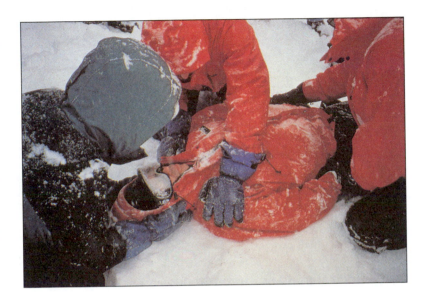

medical personnel. It also applies to group leaders, guides, and designated health providers for a group.

3. In all instances you are expected to follow accepted guidelines and act as would another prudent person with similar training under the same circumstances.

4. You are not expected to give treatment or carry out procedures for which you have not been trained.

5. Many states have "Good Samaritan" laws that protect first aiders from successful suits provided that
   • the aid is given during an emergency;
   • treatment is unscheduled, unanticipated (an emergency), and given in good faith;
   • no monetary compensation is received for providing care.
   Good Samaritan laws do not protect against gross negligence in providing care.

6. You are not expected to place your own life and safety in jeopardy.

7. Once treatment has started, you are legally bound to remain with the victim until care is turned over to an equally or better trained person or group. Otherwise leaving a victim may be interpreted as negligent abandonment, unless your own safety is threatened.

8. Obtain consent before touching a person. Usually consent is verbally expressed or implied. If a victim refuses help, try to persuade him or her to accept it. If a victim is mentally disturbed or medically incompetent (incapable of making a rational decision) and acting in a way that is detrimental to his or her health, you are legally justified in providing care. If a victim is a minor (under 18 years of age) and a parent or guardian is unavailable, consent is implied and treatment may be given. Most youth programs require pretrip signed consent from parents.

9. Explain any treatment you are about to give. If treatment involves a procedure such as reducing a dislocated shoulder, explain your training and experience.

10. Whenever possible, involve victims in discussions and decisions concerning their care.

Psychological and Emotional Issues

In a wilderness emergency, first aiders, as well as victims and bystanders, experience personal stress due to the isolation, absence of definitive medical care, pain, and difficulties of prolonged evacuation. Anxiety or panic may compromise safety and interfere with rescue and first aid. Personality traits determine how an individual reacts to such an emergency.

As a rescuer you should provide comfort and reassurance to the victim. Reducing anxiety can decrease the pain and severity of injuries by reducing muscular spasm and tension. Try to

- Discuss the victim's condition calmly and honestly.
- Encourage the victim to express his or her feelings. Listen, but do not judge.
- Give realistic answers to the victim's questions, but try to be positive.
- Explain what you are doing and why you are doing it.
- Use stress management techniques like slow, deep breathing, muscle relaxation, and imagining pleasant events or places to reduce pain and anxiety.
- Let the victim take part in the physical care and ask his or her opinion about decisions involving that care. This helps preserve the victim's dignity and self-esteem and reduces a victim's guilt that may later cause emotional disturbances.

Providing first aid is stressful for both you and the victim. You may feel frustrated by your inability to control the situation or to help; angry at the victim for interfering with your plans or at the dangers and difficulty of the rescue; and sickened by seeing serious injuries. If you feel overwhelmed, stop for a moment, calm yourself, and redirect your thoughts, or ask someone else to help you or take over.

After treating severe injuries, you may experience post-traumatic stress disorder, an emotional reaction that may include frustration, depression, and flashbacks. These reactions are now well recognized and addressed routinely by professional rescue personnel after difficult situations. To prevent later emotional problems, discuss your feelings with a trusted friend, mental health professional, or clergy within 24 to 72 hours of helping at a traumatic incident. This brings out feelings quickly and reduces personal anxieties and stress.

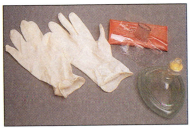

Infectious disease barriers for first aid

Infectious Disease Precautions

First-aiders risk exposure to infectious diseases when caring for victims. The most serious diseases are bloodborne, caused by microorganisms present in blood. Use protective gloves (i.e., latex) and eye, face, and mouth protection to prevent contact with blood and body fluids. Admittedly, such precautions may be difficult in many wilderness emergencies. Nonsterile protective gloves and a mouth-to-barrier device for rescue breathing should be carried in the wilderness first aid kit, as well as glasses or goggles to protect against splashing or spurting blood. A bandana can be tied over the mouth and nose to serve as a mask. However, do not delay control of serious bleeding or rescue breathing because protection is not available.

Hepatitis B and the human immunodeficiency virus (HIV) infection that causes AIDS are serious viral diseases that are spread by contact with infected blood. Other transmissible bloodborne diseases are hepatitis C, D, and E, and syphilis. Hepatitis B attacks the liver and causes jaundice, chronic illness, and occasional death. HIV disables the immune system, preventing the body from fighting off infections. Presently, AIDS is incurable and all victims eventually die from it.

Vaccines are available to prevent hepatitis B infection, but not AIDS. People infected with HIV may be unaware that they are contagious.

Because of the risk of these serious bloodborne diseases, first-aiders should treat blood and body fluids (since all body fluids may contain blood) as if they were infectious.

Try to avoid infections that are spread through the air by coughing and sneezing (e.g., tuberculosis) by using a mouth-to-barrier device for rescue breathing.

In fact, the risk of infection while giving first aid is extremely low. The risk of infection through blood splashing on a mucous membrane (eye, mouth) or exposure or contact with blood through minor scrapes on the skin is too low to be accurately measured. No cases are known of disease transmission to rescuers from giving unprotected rescue breathing to an infected victim.

After giving first aid, vigorously wash your hands and exposed skin for 15 to 20 seconds with soap, especially if they have been in contact with the victim's blood. If your mouth and/or your eyes are exposed to blood, rinse or flush them with copious amounts of water.

If exposure to blood has occurred, and especially if there has been direct contact between a victim's blood and a wound on your skin, seek medical advice later. Requesting a test of the victim's blood for HIV may be desirable but is a complicated legal matter. In most cases, such testing cannot be done without the victim's consent.

Immunizations

No special immunizations are needed for wilderness activities in North America and other developed areas. Keep routine immunizations up to date. For remote travel in less developed areas, other vaccinations may be recommended (see Table 1.1). Table 1.2 suggests resources for specific information.

Cholera immunization is not recommended for any international destination. Hepatitis B vaccination is now routinely given to infants.

Tetanus, a serious infection acquired through contamination of wounds, is rarely seen in the United States because all children are routinely immunized. Adults need a booster shot every 10 years.

Pre-exposure rabies vaccination is not needed for North America except for animal researchers or veterinarians, who could be bitten. Rabies is discussed in chapter 17.

Immunizations

TABLE 1.1

Routine	May Be Required at International Border	Commonly Recommended for International Travel	Special Needs
diphtheria, pertussis, tetanus (DPT) measles, mumps, rubella (MMR) polio	yellow fever cholera	typhoid hepatitis A	hepatitis B rabies Japanese encephalitis

Resources for Foreign Travel Immunizations

TABLE 1.2

- Current health care provider
- Local county or state health department
- U.S. Public Health Service Quarantine Stations
  Chicago, Honolulu, Los Angeles, Miami, New York, San Francisco, Seattle
- Centers for Disease Control and Prevention
  Detailed, current, recorded voice or printed fax information:
  (404) 332-4559
  Internet address: http://www.cdc.gov
- International Association for Medical Assistance to Travelers (IAMAT)
  Charts immunizations, malaria risk, lists of doctors overseas
  417 Center St., Lewiston, NY 14092; (716) 754-4883

chapter 2

Action at an Emergency

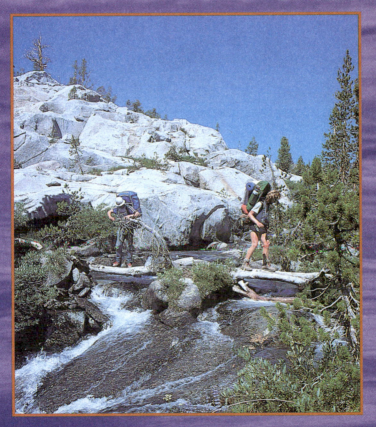

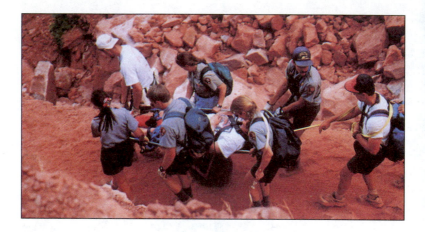

Chances are, at some time you will have to decide whether to help another person in distress. Effective action is based on pre-emergency planning and training. Information about the incident may be sketchy and inaccurate, but will probably contain something about the nature of the accident: a near drowning, an avalanche, a burn, a bad laceration. As you approach the scene, review what to do, whom to call for help, and how to contact them. You may be a member of a group going to the scene. If so, talk with the other members and decide about assigning responsibilities, because different people will have different skills. If you are one of a group that is not a formal rescue group, choose a leader to make the decisions. Try to arrive at the scene of the accident with at least a basic plan, an understanding of how you can help, and a course of action should evacuation be necessary.

Approaching a Victim
SCENE SURVEY

First, do a 10-second scene survey. Is the site safe? Is another avalanche or rockfall a possibility? Is there a dangerous animal to be avoided? Is there a spreading fire? Is the water too rough for a safe rescue?

In the first few minutes, determine the cause of the injury. The mechanism of the injury may help you to determine its extent or suspect hidden injuries.

How many people are injured?. There may be more than one victim; look for others.

You cannot help if you become a victim!

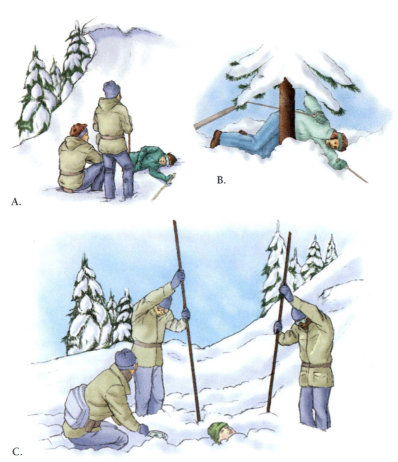

A.

B.

C.

Scene survey: Assess hazards (A), the extent and cause of injury (B), and the number of victims (C)

Mechanisms of Injury

Consideration of the mechanisms of injury will help you understand the injury and predict its severity.

Most injuries involve an impact between stationary and moving objects. A moving object develops more energy in proportion to its speed than its weight. Double the weight and the energy doubles; but double the speed and the energy increases fourfold.

At an accident scene when trying to reconstruct the event, consider the following:

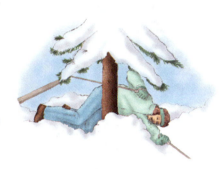

Reconstructing the accident

- What was the distance of the fall, or speed of the moving object? Were the forces involved strong enough to produce serious injuries?

- In what direction and on what body part did the forces act?

- Where would you expect to find injuries?

- Are internal injuries likely?

- Is a spinal injury likely?

Suspect multiple, serious injuries, including internal injuries, in

- a fall of 2½ to 3 times body height (big mass, relatively low speed);

- a motorcycle, all-terrain vehicle, or snowmobile accident, especially if no helmet was worn (big mass, high speed);

- a high-speed skier or snowboarder collision (big mass, high speed);

- a gunshot wound of the head, neck, or trunk (small mass, very high speed).

Getting to Victims

Do not attempt a rescue unless it can be done without endangering the rescuers. Weather, the location of the victim, avalanche danger, fire, and entrapment of the victim may all pose hazards. Specialized rescue teams may be needed.

WATER RESCUE

Reach-Throw-Row-Go is the sequence for attempting a water rescue.

Reach. First, reach for the victim with a lightweight pole, ladder, long stick, branch, or any other available object. Secure your footing and have a bystander grab your belt or pants for stability. Keep your weight low and back.

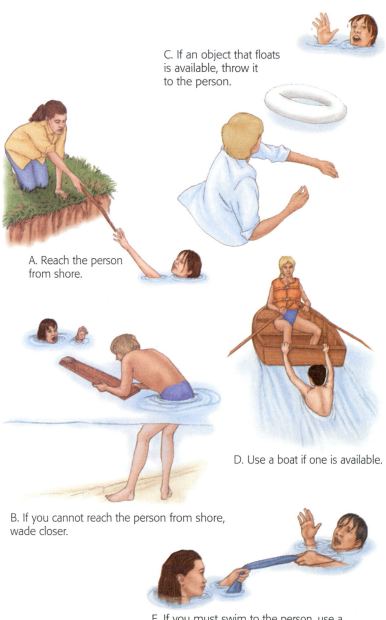

C. If an object that floats is available, throw it to the person.

A. Reach the person from shore.

D. Use a boat if one is available.

B. If you cannot reach the person from shore, wade closer.

E. If you must swim to the person, use a towel or board for him or her to hold onto. Do not let the person grab you.

Water rescue

Throw. Throw anything available that floats—empty picnic jug, empty fuel can, life jacket, floating cushion, pieces of wood, inflated spare inner tube or tire. If possible, tie a rope to the object to be thrown to pull in the victim. If you miss, you can retrieve the object and throw again. Few people can accurately throw an object farther than 50 feet.

Row. If the victim is out of range and there is a nearby rowboat, canoe, or motorboat, try rowing. Boat handling is dangerous and requires skill. Always wear a life jacket (personal flotation device, or PFD) for your own safety. To avoid capsizing, pull the victim in over the stern or bow, not over the side of the boat.

Go. Rescue a drowning victim by swimming *only if you are a strong swimmer and trained in rescue techniques.* A swimming rescue, even in calm water, is difficult and hazardous; frequently a would-be rescuer becomes a victim. If you enter the water, wear a life jacket, if available, and carry something (extra life jacket, plank) to place between you and the victim.

 DO NOT
- **try to rescue a drowning person by swimming unless you are trained in lifesaving.**

ICE RESCUE

If someone falls through ice near the shore, extend a pole or throw a line with a floating object attached. If the victim has fallen through ice far from the shore and cannot be reached with a pole or a thrown line, lie flat and push a ladder, plank, or tree limb ahead of you for the victim to grasp. Or tie a rope anchored to the shore to a spare tire; lie flat and push the tire ahead of you. Pull the victim ashore or to the edge of the ice.

Self Rescue If someone who has fallen through the ice can get his/her upper body out of the water and onto the ice, they may be able to pull forward, continuing to keep as flat as possible to spread the weight.

 DO NOT
- **go near broken ice without supporting helpers.**

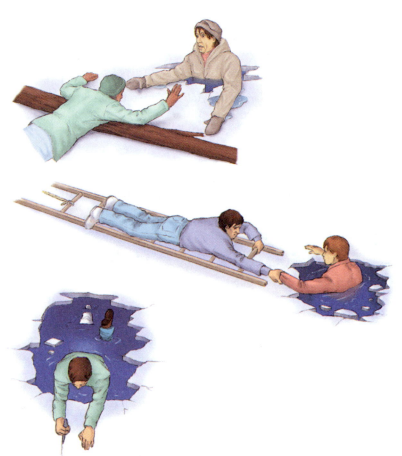

Lie flat on the ice and push a plank, ladder, or tree limb ahead of you for the victim to grasp. Pull the victim to the edge of the ice. Keep as flat on the ice as possible and pull yourself forward.

ELECTRICAL EMERGENCY RESCUE

Even mild electrical shocks can cause serious internal injuries or death. A current greater than 1000 volts is considered high voltage, but the 110 volts of household current can also be deadly.

Electricity enters the body at the point of contact and travels along the paths of least resistance (nerves and blood vessels). Current traveling through the body generates heat and destroys cells.

DO NOT

- touch an appliance or the victim until the current is off.
- try to move downed wires.
- use any object, even a dry wood broom, tool, chair, or stool, to separate the victim from a high-voltage electrical source. It will not protect you.

Low Voltage (Inside Buildings)   Most indoor electrocutions are caused by faulty equipment or careless use of appliances. Turn off the electricity at the circuit breaker, fuse box, or outside switchbox, or unplug the appliance.

High Voltage (Power Lines)   If you feel a tingling sensation in your arms, legs, or lower body, stop. Do not continue to approach the victim. This sensation signals that you may be on energized ground and that an electrical current is passing through your body. If this happens, raise one foot off the ground, turn around, and hop to a safe place. Wait for trained personnel with the proper equipment to cut or disconnect the wires.

Power Line Fallen over Vehicle   Tell the driver and passengers to stay in the vehicle. Only if an explosion or fire threatens a car should anyone try to jump out.

MOTOR VEHICLE ACCIDENTS

In most states you have a legal obligation to stop and give help when *personally* involved in a motor vehicle accident. If you come upon an accident shortly after it has happened, the law does not require you to stop, even if you see that help is needed.

What to Do

1. Stop your vehicle in a safe place. If the police are present, do not stop unless asked to do so.
2. Turn on your flashing hazard lights, place warning reflectors or warning flares.
3. Direct someone to warn other drivers.
4. Try to enter the accident vehicle through a door. If the doors are jammed, someone inside the car may be able to roll down a window. As a last resort, break a window. Once inside, place the vehicle in "park," turn off the engine, and set the parking brake.

5. Stabilize the head and neck of an unresponsive victim or one who might have a spinal injury (see chapter 11).

6. Treat life-threatening injuries.

7. Whenever possible, wait for trained emergency personnel to extricate victims.

WILDLAND FIRES

Back-country travelers and people who live in the urban-wildland interface may encounter wildland fires. They should be aware of how fires spread, the causes of injury and death, and safety measures to avoid the hazards.

Fires have three requirements: heat, oxygen, and fuel. They are, therefore, more common in hot, dry climates; are fanned into greater intensity by wind; and need trees, bushes, and grass as fuel. Intense blasts of heat can kill without direct burning. Fire spreads by direct extension and "spotting" (the spread of fire by flying, burning debris).

Be aware of the fire hazards around you. The hazards in your camp include stoves and fuel. Hazards in the environment include dry grass, flammable trees, and bushes.

Camp in safe places. Keep fire or stove sites clear of brush and dry fuel.

The safest spots near a fire are along its flanks, behind the advancing fire (upwind), and downhill rather than uphill (fires spread rapidly uphill).

Safety during a fire depends on following the **LCES** principle—Lookouts, Communication, Escape routes, Safety zones. Be constantly on the lookout for changes in the direction of the fire. Be able to communicate these changes to others. Plan your escape routes and potential safety zones.

Heart attacks and heat stress are the most common causes of death among firefighters. Internal trauma, burns, and asphyxiation account for most other deaths. Injuries include burns and trauma from falling objects.

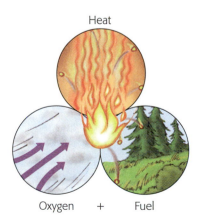

Heat

Oxygen   +   Fuel

How fires spread

What to Do

1. Get the people out fast.

2. Call for help.

3. Use an extinguisher only if the fire is small and your own escape route is clear. Fighting a fire during the first five minutes is crucial.

4. Tear burning clothing off the victim, especially away from the face. Synthetic materials—polypropylene, polyester, nylon—melt rapidly at high temperatures and cause deep, severe burns. Most of the "high tech" materials used in outdoor clothing and tents are potentially very hazardous. Some are treated with fire retardants, but all should be regarded as dangerous in fires. Remove burning fragments of these materials from the victim as rapidly as possible.

5. Throw water over the victim. Wrap a rug or blanket around the victim's neck and try to keep flames from the face. Flannel sleeping bags are safe wraps, but synthetic sleeping bags and clothing used to smother flames could melt and cause deeper burns. Roll the victim on the ground to extinguish the flames. Restrain the victim from running and fanning the flames.

 DO NOT

- **let a victim run with clothing on fire.**
- **get trapped while fighting a fire. Always keep an escape route open so you can exit rapidly.**

ANIMALS

Approach situations involving animals with caution; wild animals are potentially dangerous. Large animals do not always retreat from humans and may attack rescuers. Most smaller animals retreat from humans, but all wild animals are unpredictable and may attack even if not provoked. Be aware of the potentially dangerous animals in the area where you are traveling. Farm animals can also be dangerous.

When threatened by an animal

- Do not stare at the animal. Look down or away.

- Back away slowly.

- Speak quietly to reassure the animal.

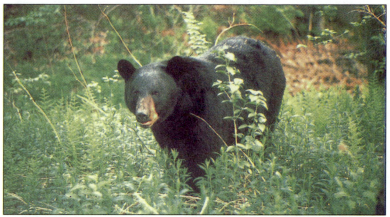

Large animals do not always retreat from humans and may attack rescuers.

If an animal has attacked another person

- Use food to lure the animal away from the victim.
- It may back off after attacking. This affords a chance to remove the victim.

Animal attacks are rare but dangerous. In general, if attacked, fight back. An exception to this recommendation is the grizzly bear and a mother black bear with her cubs. In these cases you should lie down and play dead. In bear country, make a noise as you travel, and be especially cautious if you see a mother with cubs.

CONFINED SPACES

A confined space is an area such as a tank, vessel, vat, silo, bin, vault, cave, or mine shaft that might contain a dangerous atmosphere. After an accident in a confined space

- Call for immediate help; activate the local EMS.
- Do not rush in to help; the space could be filled with toxic gas.
- When help arrives, try to rescue the victim without entering the space.
- If rescue from the outside is impossible, trained and properly equipped rescuers must enter the space to remove the victim.
- Administer first aid, rescue breathing, or CPR if necessary (see appendix A).

Moving a Victim

Do not move a victim until he or she is stable and ready for transportation. First provide all necessary first aid. Move a victim only if there is immediate danger from environmental hazards; if it is impossible to gain access to other victims (e.g., in a vehicle) who need life-saving care; or if the victim's heart has stopped, in which case move him or her to a flat, firm surface on which CPR and rescue breathing can be carried out. Move the victim if it is impossible to administer first aid at the scene.

 DO NOT

- move victims prematurely unless they are in immediate danger or must be moved to shelter while waiting for rescue.
- make an injury worse by moving the victim.
- move a victim who might have a spinal cord injury without first stabilizing the spine.
- move a victim unless you know where you are going to place him/her.
- try to move a victim by yourself if others are available to help.

EMERGENCY MOVES

Do not aggravate a spinal injury or other major injury by moving the victim too quickly. Place the victim supine. Protect the spine (see chapter 8). If time and safety permit, stabilize all injured parts before and during moving.

Drags Use a shoulder drag for carrying a victim short distances over a rough surface. Stabilize the victim's head with your forearms. Or, with a blanket pull, roll the victim onto a blanket and pull from behind the head.

NONEMERGENCY MOVES

One-Person Moves You can help a victim to walk by acting as a "human crutch": If one leg is injured, the victim can walk on the good leg while you support the injured side. Use a cradle carry for children and lightweight adults who cannot walk and in whom spinal injury is not suspected. Use a fireman's carry if the victim's injuries permit; longer distances can be traveled if the victim is carried over your shoulder. Use a piggy-back carry when the victim cannot walk but can hang onto you.

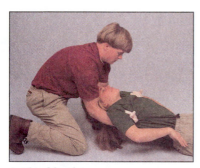

A. Shoulder drag

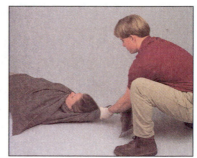

B. Blanket drag

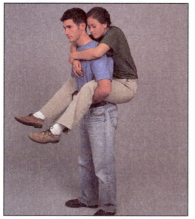

C. Piggyback

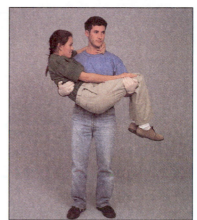

D. Cradle

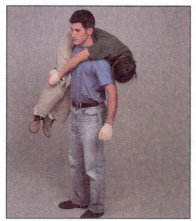

E. Fireman carry

Two-or-More-Person Moves   Two or more people can help a victim to walk by using the two-handed carry. The four-handed seat carry is the easiest two-person carry when no equipment is available; use it when the victim cannot walk but can use his/her arms to hang onto rescuers. Use an extremity carry when the victim has one injured leg but, with help, can hop for a short distance on the other leg. Use a hammock carry if three to six people can stand on alternate sides of the injured person and link hands beneath the victim.

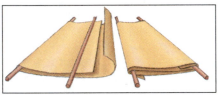

Blanket and pole stretcher

Stretcher or Litter   The safest way to carry an injured victim without a spinal injury is on a stretcher or improvised stretcher. Test improvised stretchers before use by lifting a rescuer who is about the same size as the victim. With a blanket-and-pole improvised stretcher, the victim's weight will keep the blanket from unwinding if it is properly wrapped. If you use a jacket and pole, button or zip up the jacket; invert the arms and pass poles through the

Principles of Lifting
- Do not try to handle too heavy or awkward a load—seek help.
- Use a safe grip. Use the palm of the hand rather than the fingers.
- Keep your back straight. Tighten the muscles of the buttocks and abdomen.
- Bend knees to use the strong muscles of thighs and buttocks.
- Keep your arms close to your body and elbows flexed.
- Position feet at shoulder width for balance, one in front of the other.
- When lifting, keep the victim close to your body.
  - Do not twist your back; pivot with the feet.
  - Lift slowly, smoothly, and in unison with other helpers.
- Tell the victim what you are about to do.
- Rest periodically.
- A party of 12–16 is needed to carry a victim a long distance over rough terrain.

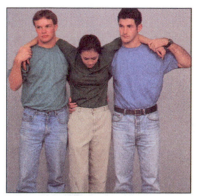

A. Two people assisting victim to walk

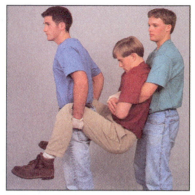

D. Extremity carry

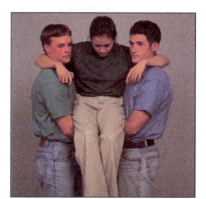

B. Two-handed seat carry

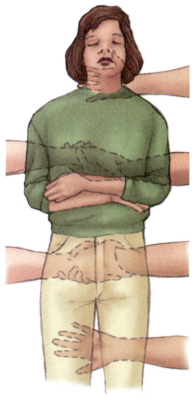

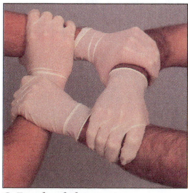

C. Four-handed seat carry

E. Hammock carry

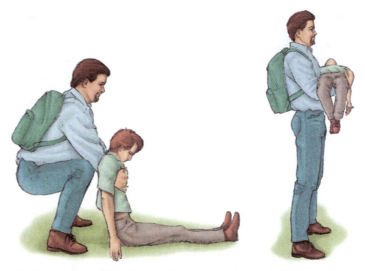

Keep back straight and bend knees. Keep victim close to body.

arm holes. A board improvised stretcher is sturdier than a blanket-and-pole stretcher but heavier and less comfortable. Secure the victim to the board. Skis, pack frames, sleds, and tree limbs can also be used to make stretchers. Pad well using sleeping bags, clothing, or sleeping pads. Commercial stretchers are seldom available except with rescue groups.

Extrication from Difficult Locations

An injured person may be thrown or fall into a site from which extrication is difficult. There are six positions in which the body can be trapped (see box below and illustration on page 27).

Basic Body Positions in Entrapment

1.   Supine, neutral position, all limbs aligned
1a. Supine, but head, back, or limbs out of alignment
2.   On side, neutral position, limbs and back aligned normally
2a. On side, but with head, back, or limbs out of alignment
3.   Prone, in neutral position, with limbs aligned
3a. Prone, but with head, back, or limbs out of alignment

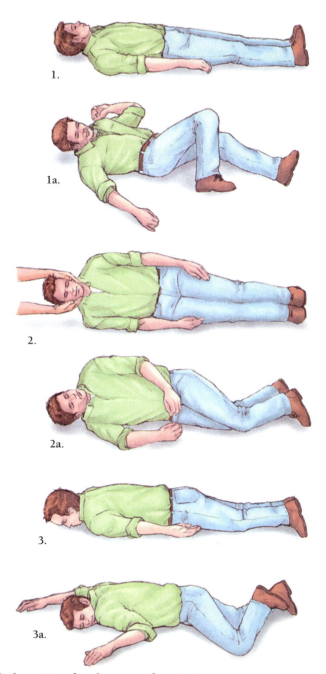

1.

1a.

2.

2a.

3.

3a.

Basic body positions found in an accident victim

Moving a victim from a position in which the body is distorted and crumpled requires skill and is not to be attempted by one person, let alone two or three people who do not know what they are doing.

Four to six experienced rescuers are needed to move a victim safely. One person in the group is designated as the leader who gives all commands. The group must lift the victim as a unit, all working simultaneously and with a clear idea of what is being attempted.

The final objective is to lay the victim flat on his/her back with the head and neck stabilized and the shoulders and hips at right angles to the vertebral column (Position 1).

Concentrate on supporting the head and neck, the shoulders, and the hips. The victim does not have to be moved from the first position into the final position in a single movement. Move in stages, lifting the victim from Position 3 to 2 to 1.

 DO NOT
- lift a victim with one person at the head and another at the feet with the victim hanging like a **U** unless you are *certain* there is *no spinal injury.*

The most difficult extraction is from a small space with limited access for rescuers. If there is any suspicion of a spinal injury, do not attempt to extract the victim. Wait for a rescue group with special equipment. Do not make matters worse than they already are. If nothing else, help the victim to keep warm and comfortable; provide food, drink, and encouragement; and get help as quickly as possible.

Seeking Help

Seeking help in the wilderness will always be difficult, and sometimes impossible where emergencies occur far from the nearest road or telephone. Before you go into a wilderness, know how to contact the local rescue group, sheriff, or police. Distance, weather, time of day, and the number of people available to go for help may limit what you do.

In the face of an emergency, **STOP**.

Stop and take a moment to calm yourself. Do not panic.

Think about the problem and the correct course of action.

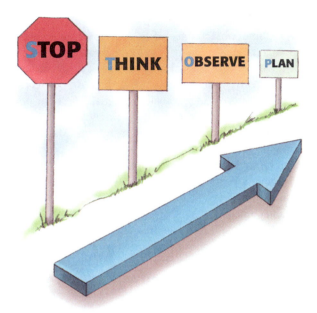

In face of emergency, **STOP.**

Observe the situation. What has occurred? What are the conditions? What resources are available?

Plan your course of action and coordinate with the other potential rescuers.

Important Planning Questions

1. Can you handle the problem in the field and let the victim continue with the trip, as with a minor wound or injury or self-limited illness? Since you may be far from help, it is reasonable to wait and observe the victim before deciding to seek help.
2. Can the person walk unaided? This may be the fastest and safest means to reach medical care—despite a painful ankle or knee injury or after a venomous snakebite.
3. Does the victim need to be carried, and do you have the resources to do this? If not, how do you get help?

If the situation is not an emergency, the victim may be able to walk out. However, if in doubt, contact medical help. If you are with a group, send a member of the party out to the nearest telephone, or, in very remote areas, try using signal mirrors, flares, or smoking fires. Many hikers now carry cellular phones, but these do not work in some areas where mountains or ridges block the signals. Cellular phones and other electronic devices should be used sparingly and ethically. Rescue groups should not be summoned for minor injuries. Many rescue groups are composed of volunteers; they must not be put to unnecessary expense or danger without good cause.

If the situation appears to be more than you can handle, contact the EMS. Use of trained rescue groups has many advantages. The emergency medical technicians (EMTs) should know what to do. In addition, they are probably in radio contact with physicians at a hospital; care provided by EMTs at the scene and on the way to the hospital can improve the victim's chances of survival and rate of recovery; emergency services have access to rapid transportation; and in some situations—cave rescue, high-angle mountain rescue—only teams with special training can rescue victims safely.

DO NOT

- rush to rescue in a dangerous situation and create more victims.
- send someone for help before assessing the victim and planning for the safety of all.
- leave injured or sick victims alone in the field, unless unavoidable.
- allow anyone to leave the group unaccompanied unless unavoidable and part of a plan.

Give the EMS the following information:

- The victim's location. Give distances from recognizable landmarks or from the nearest road; names of valleys or creeks. Compass bearings from landmarks and map coordinates are ideal.
- Your name, the name of the victim, and family contacts.
- The nature of the emergency (e.g., heart attack, drowning).
- Number of persons needing help and any special medical conditions.

- The victim's condition (conscious, breathing, fractures) and what is being done for the victim (rescue breathing, CPR).

- A description of local weather conditions if the information might affect rescue plans.

- Information about where, and if, you can be contacted; provide information about future contacts (time, frequency).

On radio or phone, speak slowly and clearly. Ask the rescuers to repeat important information. Always be the last to hang up. If you send someone to make the call, have the caller report back to you to ensure the call was made.

Each section in this book will consider criteria for evacuation of people with specific problems.

Guidelines for Evacuation
GENERAL GUIDELINES
The victim's health or survival may depend on your ability to move him/her from the scene. The following list describes conditions that may necessitate evacuation.

1. Deteriorating condition, increasing shortness of breath, altered mental status, shock, progressive weakness, persistent vomiting and/or diarrhea, inability to tolerate oral fluids, fainting when attempting to stand (see chapters 9, 10, 11, 12)

2. Severe pain

3. Inability to walk at a reasonable pace due to a medical problem

4. Severe or ongoing bleeding from any site, including wounds; blood in the vomit or stool (see chapters 4, 12)

5. Signs and symptoms of serious high-altitude illness (see chapter 15)

6. Worsening infections

7. Chest pain that is not clearly musculoskeletal in origin—possible heart attack (see chapter 9)

8. Psychological disorder that impairs the safety of the person or group

9. Near drowning (see chapter 19)

10. Large or serious wounds or burns, or wounds with particular complications, such as fractures that break the overlying skin, gunshot wounds, deformed fractures, fractures with impaired circulation, impaled objects, suspected spinal injury (see chapters 4, 8, 11)

11. Serious mechanism of injury (at least warrants close observation): fall from greater than 20 feet; motorcycle, all-terrain vehicle, or snowmobile crash; closed vehicle crash involving high speed, rollover, victim ejection, or death of another occupant; high-speed skiing collision; injury by rockfall or avalanche

Travel may continue if it is toward medical care in the case of points 3, 4, and 8, or when descending in the case of 5.*

HELICOPTER EVACUATION

Helicopters can sometimes greatly reduce the time required for an emergency transport, but create additional risks for both crew and victim. In very remote areas, it may take so long to contact the helicopter service that it is quicker to start a ground evacuation. The decision to use a helicopter for evacuation must take into account logistical and environmental factors.

Evacuate by Helicopter If:

1. a victim's life might be saved
2. the victim has a significantly better chance for full recovery with a helicopter evacuation
3. the pilot believes that weather and landing zone conditions are safe
4. ground evacuation may be dangerous or prolonged
5. not enough rescuers are available for a ground evacuation

*Adapted from the *Wilderness Medical Society Practice Guidelines for Wilderness Emergency Care.* Merrillville, IN: ISC Books, 1995.

CHAPTER 3

Victim Assessment and Urgent Care

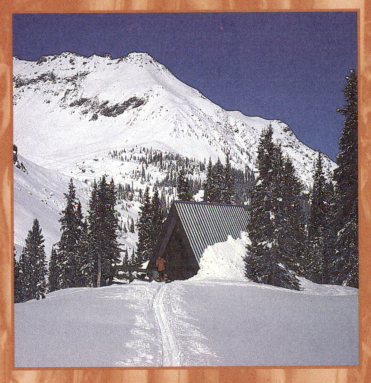

Scene Survey • Initial (Primary) Survey • Victim's History •

Vital Signs and Physical Exam • Ongoing Assessment •

Multiple Victim Incidents (Triage)

To find out what is wrong with a victim, you must be able to do a rapid, but accurate, examination, called *assessment*. In wilderness first aid, help and other resources are limited, care for serious injuries and illnesses may be primitive, and the only first aid equipment available is what you have with you or can improvise. Unlike urban first aid, there is no 911 to call, no EMTs to take over for you, and no ambulance to transport the victim. The decision, however necessary, to transport a victim to medical care cannot be made lightly, since it takes time and manpower. Therefore, the ability to find out what is occurring and its significance through the development of good assessment skills is very important.

This chapter presents a detailed and systematic method for assessing a victim and giving urgent first aid. Assessment must be learned well and practiced regularly to avoid missing important, life-threatening problems.

Assessment takes different forms, depending on whether the victim is responsive or unresponsive, injured or ill. The terms *responsive* and *unresponsive* are used instead of conscious and unconscious, since they identify what the first aider actually observes and do not require a diagnosis. Not all parts of the assessment will apply to every victim and the order of use of these parts may vary depending on the nature of the victim's problem. Most victims do not require a complete assessment. For example, a victim who cuts a finger while whittling a stick *won't* require a complete assessment, but a victim with a cut finger from slipping and falling 20 feet down a mountainside *will*, because other injuries may be present. Also, a victim may be injured and ill at the same time.

Victim assessment is divided into five parts: (1) scene survey, (2) initial survey, (3) victim's history, (4) vital signs and physical exam, and (5) ongoing assessment. Table 3.1 outlines the assessment sequences for injured and ill, responsive and unresponsive victims.

Scene Survey

The scene survey, discussed in chapter 2, gives you the first impression of what has happened and reveals hazards to the victim or yourself. Before beginning a scene survey, always protect yourself if there is a chance of contact with blood or other body fluids (see chapter 1). Put on vinyl or latex gloves before entering the scene. In cold weather, put them over a thin pair of polypropylene or silk gloves to avoid chilling your hands.

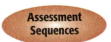

Assessment
Sequences

TABLE 3.1

Injured Victim		Ill Victim	
Unresponsive	**Responsive**	**Unresponsive**	**Responsive**
Initial/primary survey	Initial/primary survey	Initial/primary survey	Initial/primary survey
Physical exam	Physical exam Only minor injury may need to be examined	Physical exam	Medical history
Vital signs	Vital signs	Vital signs	Physical exam Only chief complaint may need to be examined
Medical history acquired from family, friends, or bystanders	Medical history	Medical history acquired from family, friends, or bystanders	Vital signs
Ongoing assessment	Ongoing assessment	Ongoing assessment	Ongoing assessment

What to Look For

➤ Is the scene safe? Check for hazards and if the scene is not safe and you cannot make it safe, do not enter.

➤ Is the victim injured or ill?

➤ If the victim is injured, what is the probable mechanism of injury?

➤ Is the victim obviously responsive or possibly unresponsive?

➤ As a general impression, does the victim appear critically injured or ill, or not?

➤ How many victims are there? For assessment and care of multiple victims, see pages 57–58.

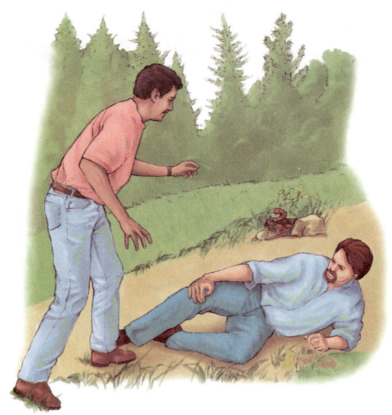

Initial assessment

Initial (Primary) Survey

Do an initial survey to detect any life-threatening conditions needing urgent care. It is important to know whether a victim is responsive or not. A responsive victim is alert, interacts with you, and knows his/her name and location. However, remember that in the wilderness it is not uncommon to lose track of the date or even day of the week. If, by the time you reach the victim, you are unsure about the level of responsiveness, tap or gently shake the victim's shoulder and ask, "Are you okay?" If the victim does not answer or the answer is garbled or unintelligible, the victim is considered unresponsive. Start immediate preparations to evacuate the victim to medical care. If other people are nearby, call for help.

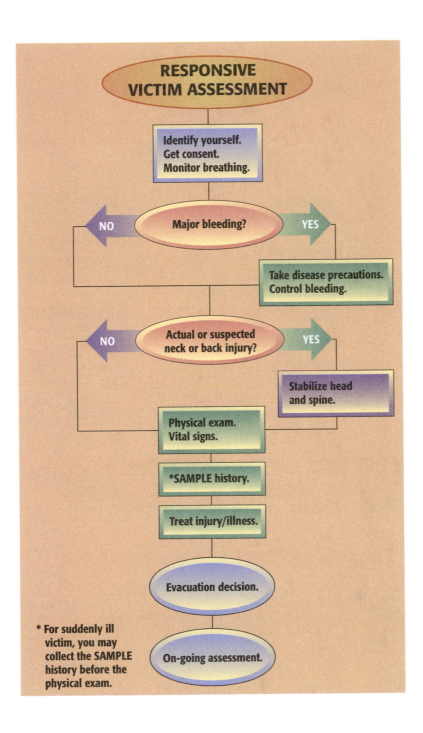

RESPONSIVE VICTIM ASSESSMENT

Identify yourself.
Get consent.
Monitor breathing.

Major bleeding?   NO   YES

Take disease precautions.
Control bleeding.

Actual or suspected neck or back injury?   NO   YES

Stabilize head and spine.

Physical exam.
Vital signs.

*SAMPLE history.

Treat injury/illness.

Evacuation decision.

On-going assessment.

* For suddenly ill victim, you may collect the SAMPLE history before the physical exam.

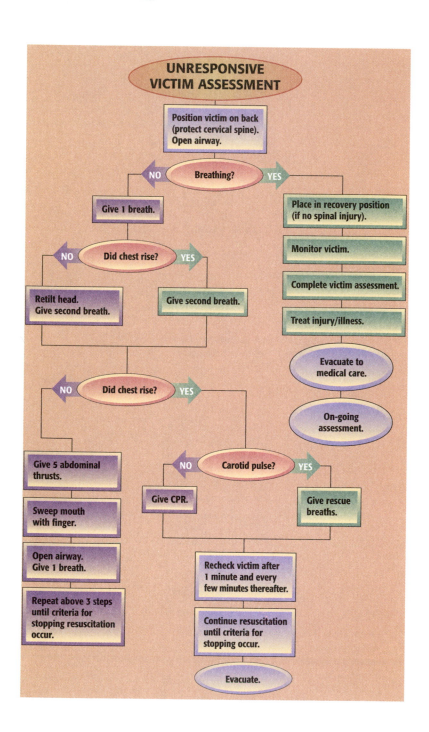

UNRESPONSIVE VICTIM ASSESSMENT

Position victim on back (protect cervical spine). Open airway.

Breathing?

NO → Give 1 breath.

YES → Place in recovery position (if no spinal injury).
→ Monitor victim.
→ Complete victim assessment.
→ Treat injury/illness.
→ Evacuate to medical care.
→ On-going assessment.

Did chest rise?

NO → Retilt head. Give second breath.

YES → Give second breath.

Did chest rise?

NO → Give 5 abdominal thrusts.
→ Sweep mouth with finger.
→ Open airway. Give 1 breath.
→ Repeat above 3 steps until criteria for stopping resuscitation occur.

YES → Carotid pulse?

Carotid pulse?

NO → Give CPR.

YES → Give rescue breaths.

Recheck victim after 1 minute and every few minutes thereafter.

Continue resuscitation until criteria for stopping occur.

Evacuate.

The initial survey assesses the respiratory and circulatory systems. A serious problem in either of these generally produces a serious threat to life. If critical problems such as abnormal breathing, an abnormal or absent pulse, or massive bleeding are identified, attend to them immediately before proceeding further. Correct problems as you find them.

Remember the first part of the initial survey by using the mnemonic **ABC.**

- **A: Airway** open?
- **B: Breathing**?
- **C: Circulation** present? Includes assessing for severe bleeding.

A: ASSESS THE AIRWAY

Unless the victim is obviously breathing normally, *immediately open the airway* with the head-tilt/chin-lift. In the unresponsive victim, the tongue and throat muscles relax so that the tongue may fall back and block the airway. The head-tilt/chin-lift brings the jaw and tongue forward and opens the airway.

What to Do

1. Place your hand nearest the victim's head on the victim's forehead. Apply backward pressure to tilt the head back.

2. Place the fingers of your other hand under the bony part of the jaw near the chin, and lift. Avoid pressing on the soft tissues under the jaw.

3. Be sure the victim's mouth remains open.

Any victim unresponsive due to an injury, especially a head injury, is assumed to have a spinal injury. In this case, do

Tongue sags and blocks airway.

Lift chin with 2-3 fingers.

Tilt head back.

Head-tilt/chin-lift

not move the victim's head or neck. Instead of the head-tilt/chin-lift, use the *jaw-thrust* maneuver:

1. Place the ring finger and little finger of each hand behind the angles of the victim's jawbone.

2. Thrust the jaw forward by lifting your hands, at the same time stabilizing the victim's head and neck with your thumbs, palms, and the index and middle fingers of each hand.

B: ASSESS BREATHING

Determine whether the victim is breathing normally, breathing inadequately, or not breathing. Place your ear over the victim's mouth and nose while keeping the airway open. Look for rise and fall of the victim's chest. Listen and feel for the movement of air.

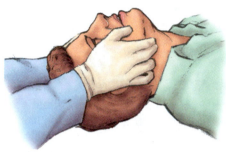

Jaw thrust

What to Do

If the victim is breathing normally, and you do not suspect a spinal injury:

1. Position the victim in the recovery position, which helps to keep the victim's tongue from falling back and blocking the airway. Vomit, if any, is more likely to be expelled than inhaled. To position an unresponsive victim who is on his/her back:

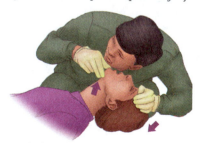

Look, listen, and feel for breathing

   • Bend the victim's left elbow to a right angle with the hand and arm still on the ground but above the head. Bend the victim's right leg so the knee is upward.

   • Place the victim's right hand against his/her left cheek with the palm facing outward. Put your right palm over the victim's right palm.

   • While keeping your palm against the victim's palm, grasp behind the victim's right bent knee and roll the victim toward you

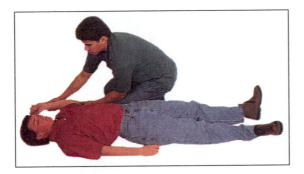

1. Bend arm. Keep legs straight.

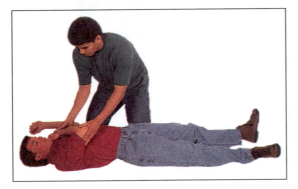

2. Place back of victim's hand against cheek and hold there.

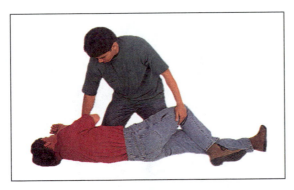

3. Hold victim's hand against cheek to support head. Pull bent leg and roll victim toward you.

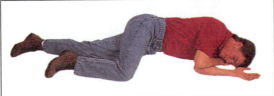

4. Front view of recovery position. Hand supports head. Bent knee prevents rolling. Bent arm gives stability.

Moving the victim into the recovery position

onto the left side. Keep the head, shoulders, and torso moving together without twisting.

- Keep the victim's right palm under the cheek to keep the head tilted and the uppermost leg bent to prevent rolling.

If the victim is not breathing:

1. Give two rescue breaths. It is very difficult to assess or care for an unresponsive victim who is lying face-down or on the side. Therefore, if not lying face-up the victim must be rolled rapidly into that position. If help is available, use a log-roll maneuver (see illustration below). If you are alone, roll the victim's body as a unit, with minimal bending or twisting of the back and neck:

- With your hand nearest the victim's head, grasp the victim's neck just below the back of the head.
- With your other hand, grasp the edge of the victim's outside hip or clothing over the edge of the hip.
- Gently roll the victim *toward* you.

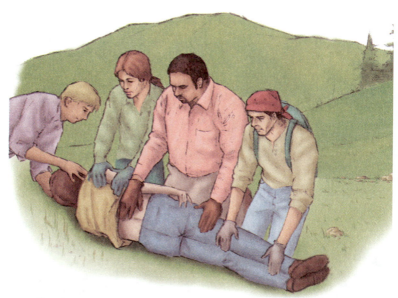

Log-roll technique

To give rescue breaths:

1. Keep the airway open with head-tilt/chin-lift (if spinal injury is suspected, use either jaw-thrust or chin-lift).

2. Pinch the victim's nose shut.

3. To protect yourself against the victim's saliva, use a mouth-to-barrier device (face shield or face mask) if available.

4. Take a deep breath and seal your lips tightly around the victim's mouth or the mouthpiece of the barrier device.

5. Give 2 slow breaths, each lasting 1½ to 2 seconds (count "one and two" at a normal speaking rate). Take a breath for yourself after each breath given to the victim.

If the first breath does not go in, reopen the airway and try another breath. If still unsuccessful, suspect foreign body airway obstruction (use *Unconscious Adult Foreign Body Airway Obstruction* procedures in appendix A).

After the rescue breaths have been given, if the victim still does not breathe or is breathing inadequately, assist breathing with mouth-to-mouth (or preferably mouth-to-barrier device). Inadequate breathing means very shallow breathing or a breathing rate that is slower than normal.

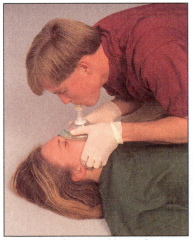 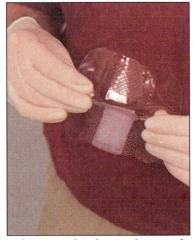

Two types of barrier devices for rescue breathing: mouth-to-barrier device and face shield

Normal breathing rates are:

- 12–20 per minute in adults and older children
- 15–30 per minute in younger children (age 1–8 years)
- 20–50 per minute in infants (under 1 year)

Assisted breathing (rescue breathing) should be at a rate of at least:

- 12 per minute in adults and older children (1 breath every 5 seconds)
- 20 per minute in younger children and infants (1 breath every 3 seconds)

Breathe into victim for 1½ to 2 seconds, then count "one-one thousand, two-one thousand," then take a deep breath before giving another rescue breath. Doing this helps give 1 breath every 5 seconds.

C: ASSESS CIRCULATION

Assessing circulation consists of checking the pulse and looking for hemorrhage (major bleeding).

What to Do

Check Carotid Artery Pulse

1. Maintain head-tilt with your hand nearest the victim's head on the forehead.

2. Locate Adam's apple with 2 or 3 fingers of your other hand.

3. Slide your fingers into the groove on the side of the Adam's apple.

4. Feel for the carotid artery pulse (take 5–10 seconds). If you suspect hypothermia, take 30 to 45 seconds to check the pulse because it may be very slow.

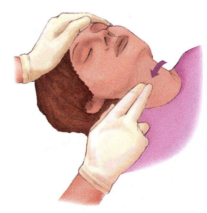

Assessing the carotid pulse

If there is a pulse but no breathing:

Give rescue breathing as described above. Every minute (12 breaths, or 1 every 5 seconds, for adults and older children, 20 breaths, or 1 every 3 seconds for young children and infants), stop to see if the victim has started to breathe spontaneously and check the pulse to see if it is still present. Continue rescue breathing until:

- Victim starts breathing on his/her own.
- Trained help, such as someone with equal or more advanced training, arrives to help you.

OR

- You are completely exhausted.

If there is no pulse, start CPR immediately! (See appendix A.)

Check for Hemorrhage Severe bleeding, either external or internal, can also be life-threatening, since a victim can bleed to death within minutes from an injury to a large artery. Check for severe bleeding by quickly looking over the entire body for blood (blood-soaked clothing, blood spurting or flowing from a wound, and/or blood pooling on the ground). If you find blood, immediately expose the suspected body area by moving, removing, or cutting clothing and find the bleeding source. Avoid contact with the victim's blood, if possible, by using vinyl or latex gloves or extra layers of cloth or dressings, and by wearing glasses or goggles and water-resistant clothing. To control bleeding, apply direct pressure over the bleeding area.

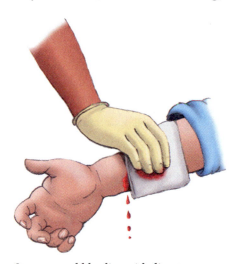

Stop external bleeding with direct pressure

Victim's History

Use the mnemonic **SAMPLE** to remember the steps in obtaining the victim's history. The best person to give the history is the victim. If the victim is unresponsive or unable to cooperate, some or all of the history can be obtained from companions. Also, ask about and look for medical-alert tags (see page 47). If you find no tags, check an unresponsive victim's wallet or purse for special medical-alert cards (have a witness present before you do this).

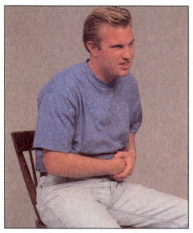

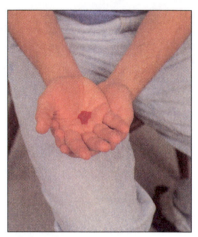

Symptom: condition described by
victim, such as abdominal pain

Sign: condition or injury
displayed, such as blood

S: Signs and Symptoms. What signs and symptoms accompany the
present event? A sign is an objective problem that you find during assessment. A symptom is a subjective problem that the victim notices
and describes to you. The signs and symptoms of various injuries are
given in detail in later chapters.

A: Allergies. Find out about any allergies to medicines, foods, insect
stings, and so on. The problem might be related to an allergic reaction.

M: Medications. Is the victim taking any prescription or nonprescription medicines (or illegal drugs)? If so, find out why the victim is taking
the medication(s).

P: Past relevant medical history. Find out about pre-existing significant
conditions, such as diabetes, heart disease, or high blood pressure.
These conditions may be contributing to the current problem. Is the
victim seeing a physician for any medical condition?

L: Last oral intake. When was the victim's last ingestion of food or
drink? It is important to know if the victim's condition is related to dehydration, weakness from lack of food, or a complication of diabetes
(see chapter 13).

E: Events leading up to the injury or illness. Find out whether anything
unusual occurred before the victim became ill or injured.

Finally, ask, "Is there anything else that I should know?"

Vital Signs and Physical Exam

The vital signs you assess include: level of responsiveness, pulse, breathing, body temperature, and skin condition. Always check vital signs at the start of a physical exam. Assess vital signs frequently during the assessment and first aid of an unstable or seriously ill or injured victim. A victim is unstable if:

- the victim's vital signs and/or mental status are abnormal and/or changing, and/or
- the victim has obvious serious injuries and/or mechanism of injury suggests that multiple and/or serious injuries may have occurred, or
- the victim appears seriously ill.

Assess vital signs occasionally in a stable victim or one with a minor illness or injury. A victim is stable if:

- the victim's vital signs and mental status are normal and unchanging, and
- the victim has no obvious serious injuries or illness and the mechanism of injury (pages 13–14) does not suggest that multiple and/or serious injuries may have occurred.

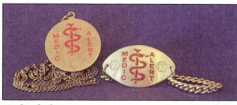

Medical-alert tags

LEVEL OF RESPONSIVENESS

A method commonly used to grade the level of responsiveness is called the **AVPU** scale:

A: Alert. Victim talks coherently, knows his or her name, address, phone number, location, and the day and date.

V: Voice. Victim is not alert, the eyes do not open spontaneously, but the victim responds in some way when you speak (stirs, moans, opens eyes).

P: Pain. Victim moves or responds in some way to a gentle but firm pinching of the skin (stirs, moans, withdraws arm or leg).

U: Unresponsive. Victim doesn't respond to voice or to pain (skin pinch over the collarbone).

Record the letter (A, V, P, or U) that corresponds to the victim's condition each time you assess the level of responsiveness.

PULSE

Place your index and middle fingertips 2 inches above the base of the thumb (radial pulse) or just to the side of the Adam's apple in the neck (carotid pulse). Generally, use the radial pulse of a responsive victim and the carotid pulse of an unresponsive or critical victim. Do not press too hard or press on both carotid arteries at the same

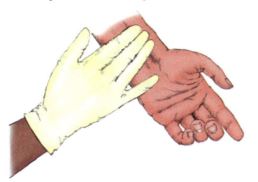

time. Repeatedly practice finding the radial and carotid pulses on yourself and your companions until you can find them easily and quickly. Count the beats for 30 seconds and multiply by 2 to get the pulse rate in beats per minute.

Assessing the radial pulse

Normal pulse rates are:

- For adults and older children: 60–100 beats/minute (as low as 50/minute may be normal for a well-conditioned athlete)
- For children (age 1–8 years): 80–100 beats/minute
- For toddlers: 100–120 beats/minute
- For infants: 120–140 beats/minute

BREATHING

Count the number of breaths for 30 seconds and multiply by 2 to obtain the breaths per minute. As you count the breaths, listen for abnormal sounds such as:

- snoring or stridor (high-pitched noises when breathing in). If present, you need to recheck the airway—it may need repositioning!
- wheezing (high-pitched noises when breathing out): Narrowing of the small air passages, as in asthma, bronchitis, or pulmonary edema. Inquire about a history of asthma, emphysema, or heart disease.

- gurgling or rattling: Material in the airway that may be causing partial blockage, such as blood, mucus, vomit, etc.

TEMPERATURE

The body temperature may alert you to fever, heat illness, or hypothermia. Measure body temperature with a thermometer placed under the tongue for 3 minutes with the lips tightly closed or in the rectum for 3 minutes. In small children or disoriented adults, put the thermometer in the armpit for at least 5 minutes. Don't use a glass thermometer when the victim is struggling or there is a chance that the victim will bite it. Rectal temperatures are the most accurate but are difficult to take, especially in bad weather.

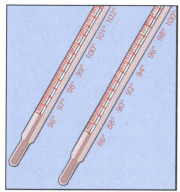

Normal and low-reading mercury thermometers

Normal body temperature is 98.6°F (range 97°–99°F) when measured by mouth. Normal rectal temperature is 99.6°F; normal axillary (armpit) temperature is 97.6°F. Carry a thermometer in your first aid kit; in cold weather it should be a special low-reading one. Mercury thermometers are the most practical type in the wilderness; alternatives are electronic thermometers designed to measure the temperature in the ear canal, mouth, or rectum. If a thermometer is unavailable, you can estimate the body temperature by putting the back of one hand (not the fingertips) on the victim's forehead (or, preferably, abdomen inside the shirt) and comparing it with your own skin temperature obtained at the same location. In a cold environment, the temperature of exposed skin is an unreliable indicator of body temperature.

SKIN CONDITION

Assess the color, temperature, and moisture of the skin.

Color and Temperature   Skin color, especially in light-skinned persons, depends on the skin circulation and the amount of oxygen in the blood. In darkly pigmented people, changes may not be apparent in the skin; therefore, examine the linings of the mouth and eyelids (mucous membranes). In a hot environment, the skin becomes warm and pink because blood flow to the skin has increased in order to lose excess heat. Hot red skin is also seen in fever and heatstroke. In a cold environment, the skin becomes cool, pale, or bluish because blood flow to the skin has decreased in order to conserve heat. Cool, cold or pale, bluish skin is seen in hypothermia, shock, and severe injuries and illnesses without fever.

Moisture   Except when wet with water, moist skin is due to sweating. Sweating occurs when the body needs to lose excess heat by evaporation, as in exercise or hot weather, or due to serious illness or injury, pain, or strong emotion, which stimulate the nervous system to activate the sweat glands.

PHYSICAL EXAMINATION

After completing the initial survey, attending to any life-threatening problems, obtaining the SAMPLE history, and checking the vital signs, make a thorough, systematic physical assessment of the victim. If possible, do this in shelter where clothing can be removed as necessary. You may discover additional problems that may not pose an immediate threat to life, but might if they remain uncorrected. Even minor injuries need care, but first they must be found.

Victims with minor injury or illness may not require a complete physical assessment. In these cases, you may examine only the injured area.

Always assess the victim's body in the following order: head, neck, chest, abdomen, extremities, and back, so that you don't forget to check an area. In inclement weather, expose only a small area of the body at a time. Use your natural tools: your eyes, ears, fingers, nose, and voice—plus your brain to evaluate what you find.

The mnemonic **DOTS** helps you remember what to look and feel for:

D: Deformities.   Compare injured and uninjured parts.

O: Open wounds.   This includes abrasions, lacerations, cuts, punctures, avulsions, and amputations. Bleeding may or may not be present.

T: Tenderness

S: Swelling

Head   Look and use both hands to feel for DOTS on the face and scalp. Look for blood or clear fluid (cerebrospinal fluid) draining from nose, ears, or mouth. Clear fluid can indicate a serious skull or spinal injury. Quickly look inside the mouth for wounds, bleeding, secretions, broken teeth, vomit, and dentures. Do not move the victim's head.

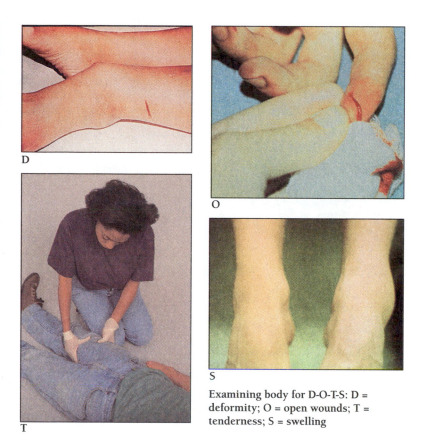

D

O

S

T

Examining body for D-O-T-S: D = deformity; O = open wounds; T = tenderness; S = swelling

Look at the pupils for reactivity, and equal size. Cover the victim's eye with your hand for 5 seconds and then uncover the eye to determine if the pupil constricts (get smaller) in response to light or the shine of a flashlight beam. Unequal pupils occur normally in a small percent of people. In a victim with a head injury, unequal pupils may mean bleeding or swelling inside the skull. Listen for abnormal noises in the nose or throat, such as gurgles, wheezes, and crowing. Smell the breath for unusual odors, such as alcohol and the fruity smell of diabetic acidosis (see chapter 13).

Neck   Look and feel for DOTS and for the popping or crackling of air under the skin from an injury to the airway. Remember, if the victim is unresponsive due to injury or if you suspect spinal injury, do not move the victim's head and neck. Look for a medical-alert tag on a chain around the neck.

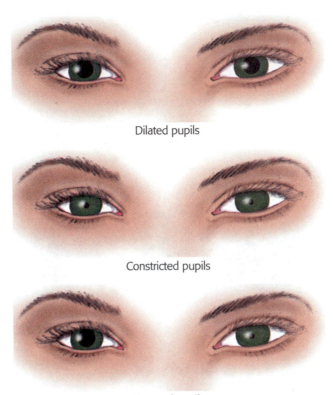

Dilated pupils

Constricted pupils

Unequal pupils

Pupils: dilated pupils, constricted pupils, unequal pupils

Chest   Look and feel for DOTS. Place one hand on each side of the chest to see whether both sides are expanding equally with inhalation. Gently squeeze both sides of the rib cage together. If this causes any pain, suspect a rib injury. Examine coughed-up material for blood or pus (yellow or green material).

Abdomen and Pelvis   Make sure your hands are warm. Using the pads of your fingertips, examine the four quadrants of the abdomen in a clockwise manner. Look and feel for DOTS, and feel gently for masses and tightening of the abdominal muscles as well as tenderness. The abdomen is normally soft. A hard or rigid area may indicate a problem.

Extremities   Compare the extremities. It is difficult to expose the thighs, legs, and arms adequately in victims wearing several layers of clothing, but these can be examined through the clothing and by

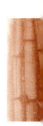

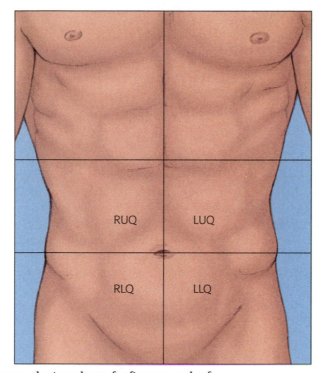

Gently press the 4 quadrants for firmness and softness

pulling clothing up or down. Look and feel for DOTS in all four extremities. Press gently with both of your hands around the arm or leg along the entire length of each extremity. If abnormalities are found and a significant injury is suspected, remove clothing over the area, using scissors or a knife if necessary, to allow direct inspection. However, *in inclement weather, do not destroy clothing that will be needed later.* Check each extremity for a pulse, sensation, and movement. Use the radial pulses for the upper extremities. Although pulses are hard to feel in the lower extremities, you may be able to feel a pulse beat in the groove behind the inner ankle bone. Pinch the skin of each forearm and leg to see if the victim reacts by telling you, moaning, or withdrawing the extremity. Look for a medical-alert bracelet.

Back   If the victim is found face-down or on the side, check the back before turning him/her face-up. If found face-up, the victim can be rolled to the side for back assessment (see log-roll, p. 42). Look and feel for DOTS. Feel the spine of each vertebra from above, moving downward. Tenderness and a "step" type of irregularity may mean a spine fracture.

Once the initial survey, history, and physical exam are completed, you will probably have a good idea of what is wrong with the victim. Suspect a spinal injury (as well as a head injury) in any unresponsive person injured in a high-velocity episode such as a motor vehicle crash; ski, mountain biking, or climbing accident; or a fall of 3 times or more the victim's height. Such accidents frequently injure the neck and/or back. If you suspect such injury, do not move the victim without using proper techniques. Avoid twisting or bending the neck or back (see chapter 11). If enough help is available, stabilize the victim's head and neck with your hands. You can also kneel with your knees on either side of the victim's head (this prevents back cramps from bending over and holding the victim's head for a long period of time). If you are alone, pack available materials around the head and neck, for example, the victim's boots, large rocks padded with clothing, or backpacks.

To do an initial survey of a responsive victim, survey the scene, approach the victim, make eye contact, and, if the victim is a stranger, introduce yourself, ask for the victim's name, and ask if you can be of help. If the victim assents, ask, "What happened to you?" The answer to this question will tell you whether the victim is injured or ill.

In the case of an injury, ask, "Do you hurt anywhere?" and ask the victim to describe what happened in detail so that you can consider the mechanism of injury. In the case of an illness, question the victim in

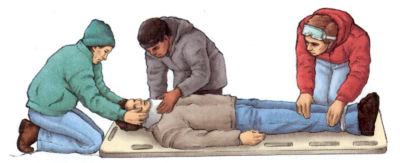

Manual stabilization of head and neck

detail regarding the signs and symptoms. The answer to these preliminary questions is called the "chief complaint." After discussing the chief
complaint, obtain a SAMPLE history from the victim (see pages 45–46).

The **ABC**s also apply to the *responsive* victim:

A: Airway open? If the victim is able to talk, the airway is open. If the
victim is choking, use techniques for obstructed airway in appendix A.

B: Breathing? If the victim is having trouble breathing, or if there are
abnormal sounds during breathing such as wheezes, gurgles, or stridor,
use the jaw-thrust maneuver to open the airway wider and/or have the
victim sit up if possible. If this doesn't work, do a quick physical exam
to look for such things as neck or chest injury and hemorrhage.

C: Circulation present? A victim must have a pulse to be responsive.
Check the radial pulse in the wrist, 2 inches above the base of the
thumb, for rate, regularity, and strength (for normal pulse rates, see page
48). Look at the ground and on the victim's clothing for signs of blood.

If in doubt about a pulse, compare it to your own or that of another
healthy person. Remember that excitement, anxiety, and pain also can
cause a fast pulse.

In the case of injury, after you have obtained the chief complaint
and assessed the ABCs, ask the victim these additional questions:

- Did you hit your head, neck, or back?
- Does your head, neck, or back hurt? Any pain anywhere else? If the
  head was injured, ask, "Were you knocked out?" If the neck or back
  was injured, ask about weakness, numbness, burning, tingling, or
  "electric-shocklike pains," especially in the arms and legs.
- Can you feel your feet?
- Can you move your feet? Ask the victim to wiggle the toes and push
  the foot down and pull it up against your hand.
- Can you feel your fingers?
- Can you move your fingers? Ask the victim to squeeze both your
  hands.

Weakness or inability to perform the above actions may indicate an
injury to the extremity or to the spinal cord. If you suspect a spinal injury, instruct the victim not to move while you are performing the rest
of the initial survey. Or, if help is available, the victim's head and neck
can be stabilized manually while the examination proceeds.

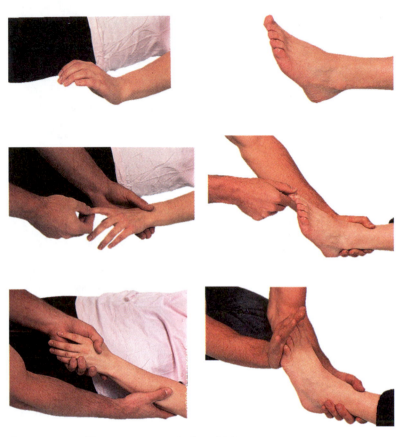

Assessing possible extremity or spinal cord injury

Next, assess the chief site of trouble indicated by the victim during the chief complaint. This should be done as described above under Physical Examination, on page 50. Assess every body area indicated by the victim as a site of pain or other abnormality. When you think you're finished, always ask the victim, "Is there anything else wrong?"

If the victim appears seriously ill or injured, if pulse or breathing is abnormal, if the mechanism of injury makes you suspect a serious injury, or if you are uneasy about the victim, proceed quickly to assessment of the vital signs and the physical exam. In good weather, remove the victim's clothing as necessary for an accurate assessment. In bad weather, assess the victim with his/her clothes on, pulling garments up or down briefly as needed. A more thorough examination can be done after shelter is reached.

To summarize, in *every* body area, look for DOTS. Also check for closed wounds, discharges, and changes in skin color. Listen for coughing and abnormal breathing sounds, such as wheezes, crows, rattles, squeaks, and stridor. Feel for tenderness, swellings, lumps, depressions, deformities, the popping feel of air under the skin in the neck and chest, and the grating sensation at an injury site that may mean a fracture. Ask the victim about pain, tenderness, inability to move, numbness, or abnormal sensations such as "pins and needles" and to squeeze both your hands simultaneously and to move all four extremities.

Compare each body area with the same area on the opposite side of the body to determine any differences. Think about the information you are gathering. What you may find and what to do will be discussed in later chapters.

Ongoing Assessment

The ongoing assessment monitors the victim's condition, which is very important when the victim is hours or days from medical care. In both injuries and illnesses, determine if the victim's condition is staying the same, getting worse, or getting better, and whether any new signs and/or symptoms are developing. Reassess the ABCs, mental status (AVPU scale), and vital signs periodically (every 15 minutes) in stable victims and more frequently (at least every 5 minutes) in unstable victims. Monitor the results of your first aid care. Calm and reassure the victim. Keep a written record of what you find!

Multiple Victim Incidents (Triage)

You may encounter emergency situations with two or more victims. This is often the case in avalanche accidents and other natural disasters. After making a quick scene survey, you must decide who is to be cared for and evacuated first. When limited personnel do not allow everything to be done right away for every victim, be guided by the principle "do the greatest good for the greatest number." This process of prioritizing victims is called "triage," a French word meaning "to sort." Note: victims of lightning strikes and other electrical accidents are exceptions to this triage procedure because of their more favorable outlook if CPR is started immediately (see appendix A). Such victims who are not breathing or do not have a pulse are classified Priority 1 and given immediate rescue breathing or CPR.

A variety of systems has been used to identify care and evacuation priorities. To find those needing immediate care for life-threatening conditions, first tell all victims who can get up and walk to move to a specific area. Victims who can get up and walk rarely have life-threatening injuries. These "walking wounded" are classified "lowest priority." Do not force a victim to move if he/she complains of pain.

Find the life-threatened, or highest-priority, victims by performing only the initial or primary survey on all remaining victims. Go to motionless victims first. You must move rapidly (spend less than 60 seconds with each victim) from one victim to the next until all have been assessed. You should not become involved in treating victims at this point, but ask knowledgeable bystanders to care for those in the highest-priority category.

Victims are placed into one of three categories:

1. Highest priority
   • Airway and breathing difficulties
   • Uncontrolled or severe bleeding
   • Decreased mental status

2. Second priority
   • Burns without airway problems
   • Major or multiple painful, swollen, deformed extremity injuries
   • Spinal injuries

3. Lowest priority
   • Minor painful, swollen, deformed extremity injuries
   • Minor soft tissue injuries
   • Death

Reassess victims regularly for changes in their condition. Only when those in the highest priority have received care should those with less serious conditions be given care.

Later, if higher-trained emergency personnel arrive on the scene, you may then be asked to continue giving first aid or help with evacuation.

This chapter introduced you to victim assessment. This process identifies information about the victim's condition: initial/primary survey, physical exam, vital signs, medical history, ongoing assessment, and multiple victim situations. Since there are four victim conditions—injured or ill responsive victims and injured or ill unresponsive victims—the sequencing of the steps varies. Without an accurate victim assessment, such as the one found in this chapter, inappropriate first aid results. Performing a good victim assessment is the mark of a good first-aider.

CHAPTER 4

Care of Bleeding, Wounds, and Burns

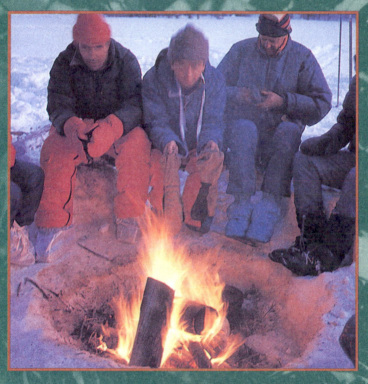

Bleeding • Wounds • Wound Care • Burns

The objectives of first aid wound care are to control bleeding, prevent infection, and protect with appropriate bandaging (see chapter 5). If kept clean, wounds are not likely to get infected and a laceration can be closed several days later, if necessary. Minor wounds do not require immediate evacuation from the wilderness.

Bleeding

The first priority of wound care is to control active bleeding.

What to Do

1. Wash your hands with soap and water before caring for a wound.

2. Put on latex gloves to protect against bloodborne infections. If gloves are unavailable, cover hands with plastic bags or similar waterproof material. You can even have the victim put pressure on a bleeding wound. After unprotected contact with blood, and after removing gloves, wash your hands vigorously with soap and water.

3. Ask the victim to sit or lie down. Fainting reactions are common after any injury, even minor wounds. Treatment increases pain and the risk of fainting, which may be mistaken for shock. If there is large blood loss, anticipate shock and treat by raising the victim's legs 8 to 12 inches. Keep the person warm.

4. Expose the wound. Because clothing may be essential for protection, do not cut garments unless absolutely necessary.

5. Place a sterile gauze pad or clean cloth directly over the entire wound, and press evenly for 5 to 10 minutes. Direct pressure stops almost all bleeding. Wounds of the scalp, hands, and face bleed more profusely because of their rich blood supply.

6. If bleeding is from an extremity, elevate the injured area above the level of the heart to reduce blood flow while continuing to apply direct pressure on the bleeding site.

7. If bleeding persists after maintaining pressure on the wound for at least 10 minutes, press harder over a wider area.

8. Apply a pressure dressing. This will allow you to attend to other injuries or victims. Make a pressure dressing by covering the wound with a thick layer of gauze or the cleanest material available, then tightly wrap a bandage over the dressing, extending above and below the site. If a pressure dressing is required, leave it in place for several hours to prevent recurrent bleeding.

Bleeding control

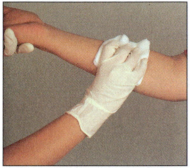

1. Direct pressure stops most bleeding.

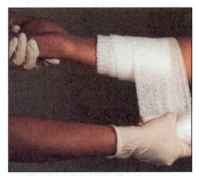

2. A pressure bandage frees you to attend to other injuries.

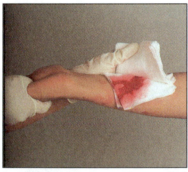

3. Add more dressings to those soaked with blood.

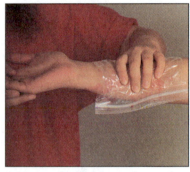

4. Use another barrier, such as a plastic bag, extra dressings or cloth, if gloves are not available.

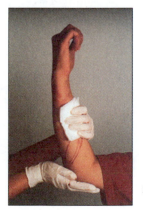

5. Use elevation to reduce blood flow if bleeding persists.

DO NOT

- apply pressure bandages so tightly that they cut off blood flow. Pain, coldness, and color change beyond the dressing suggest the bandage is too tight.
- use pressure points to control bleeding; they are difficult to find. Direct pressure should be effective.
- apply a tourniquet. The only exception may be an amputated limb or a gunshot wound with profuse bleeding. Then the tourniquet should be applied just above the amputation. It should be made of broad, flat material such as a scarf or wide belt and should not be released until the person is in the hands of a physician. Tourniquets shut off blood supply and can cause the loss of an arm or leg.
- apply pressure to control bleeding from an eyeball injury (use pressure only on wounds of the eyelids or around the eye). Avoid pressure on a wound with an embedded object or with bone protruding. In these cases, use a doughnut-shaped pad that applies pressure around the wound instead of directly on it.

Wounds

TYPES OF WOUNDS

Abrasions (scrapes, "road rash," and "rug burn") result in partial loss of the skin surface. They usually produce little bleeding but are very painful. *Lacerations* are cut skin with jagged edges. They can cause major bleeding and involve other structures below the skin such as tendons, nerves, and large blood vessels. *Incisions* are smooth-edged cuts. *Puncture wounds* are produced by pointed objects such as nails or knives that leave small entry wounds, may extend deeply, and have the greatest risk of infection. The object that produces the injury, or other foreign matter, may still be in the wound. *Avulsions* are tearing wounds that create a flap of skin and tissue still attached by a bridge of skin. *Amputations* result when a part of the body is completely separated from the body.

Wound Care
What to Do

1. Clean the wound. Although cleaning may restart bleeding, it is essential.

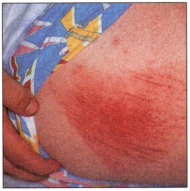

Abrasion

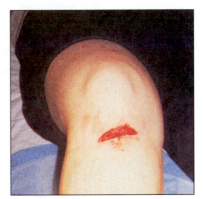

Knee laceration

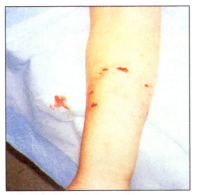

Puncture (dog bite)

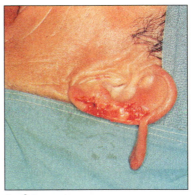

Avulsion

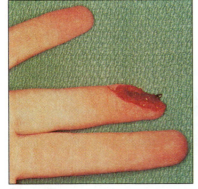

Amputation

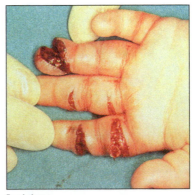

Incision

2. For a shallow wound, wash the inside of the wound and surrounding skin with soap and clean water.

3. Cover the wound with a sterile or clean dressing.

4. Flush the wound with disinfected water (see appendix B for water treatment).

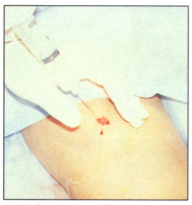

Wound irrigation

WOUND IRRIGATION

Using a large syringe (20 cc) held just above the wound, squirt water forcefully into the depths of the wound. Wear glasses or shield your face with a hand to prevent splashing of blood into your eyes and mouth. Spread the wound open so that the fluid can reach the depths of the wound. Flush out small pieces of foreign matter. Continue irrigating well after all foreign material, clotted blood, and loose tissue fragments seem to have been removed. Forceful irrigation is painful but essential for a dirty laceration.

A bulb syringe or a plastic bag with a small hole in the corner does not provide enough forceful pressure. Pouring water on a wound or soaking the wound are not satisfactory substitutes for forceful irrigation.

Remove remaining fragments with tweezers (after sterilizing the tips with a flame) or use clean gauze to wipe out embedded dirt, then irrigate again.

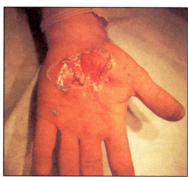

Dirty abrasion

Do not put disinfectants, such as rubbing alcohol, iodine, povidone-iodine, mercurochrome or merthiolate, or 3% hydrogen peroxide in the wound. Use them to clean the skin *around* the wound. Although commonly used, such agents are not needed; they may harm tissue and delay healing.

If the wound is an abrasion, wash, rubbing gently to remove dirt. Cover with a thin layer of antibiotic ointment, a nonstick dressing, and a bandage or tape. Shallow wounds can be covered by a thin layer of antibiotic ointment.

In the event of a small puncture wound, clean only the surface, not the depths of the wound. Encouraging bleeding is not beneficial.

EVALUATING FUNCTION

Check for normal movement and sensation beyond the wound, especially with wounds on or near the hands and feet or other joints. If a tendon in the hand is cut, the victim cannot move the finger. Manage the wound the same, but splint the finger. The tendon can be repaired days later.

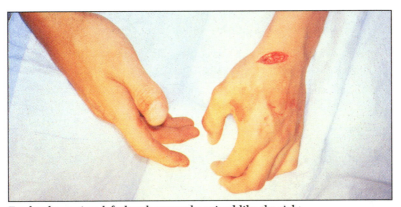

Tendon laceration: left thumb cannot be raised like the right

WOUND CLOSURE

Close small, clean wounds with tape or "butterfly" strips if the edges can be pulled together easily. Do not suture wounds. For a forehead laceration as shown, tie the hair across the scalp wound and use tape strips to close. Bandage as shown on page 86. Pack large gaping wounds and

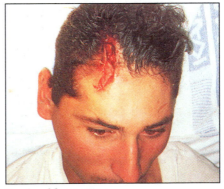

Forehead laceration

dirty wounds with sterile dressings held in place by a bandage; change daily until seen by a physician. Wounds can be sutured 3 to 5 days later.

Wilderness Tip

Scalp wounds can be closed by wetting and twisting small bundles of hair on either side of the wounds and tying them across the wound.

What to Do

Close a wound with strips of tape—"butterfly bandages."

1. Fashion strips by cutting the corners off a folded piece of ½" or 1" tape, or tear or cut tape vertically to obtain strips about ¼" wide.

2. Unfold and apply tape to one side of wound. (If you have benzoin in first aid kit, apply it to the skin first and wait about 30 seconds until it becomes sticky.) Squeeze the wound together and tape across the other side.

3. Apply strips ¼" to ½" apart. Secure the ends with perpendicular strips of tape.

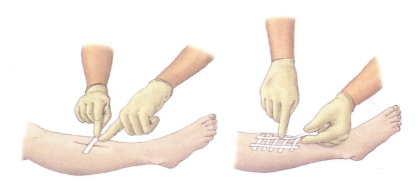

Tetanus

Tetanus ("lockjaw") causes spasm of the jaw muscles, as well as other symptoms. It is caused by a toxin produced by bacteria that enter the body through wounds. The bacterial spores are hardy and widespread in the environment, especially in areas with animal droppings. Neither the infection nor the toxin is spread from one person to another. Immunization is highly effective, but only when given before or within 72 hours after an injury. Immunization against tetanus is usually given in childhood, but boosters are needed every 10 years. People who have had routine childhood vaccinations but no boosters within the past 10 years do not need to worry after a minor cut, scratch, or bite; they should seek medical advice after returning. Large and deep wounds contaminated with dirt may warrant earlier immunization, but the victim would usually be evacuated for these injuries anyway.

Tetanus immunization is needed by

- anyone with a wound who has never been immunized against tetanus
- anyone who has been immunized but has not received a tetanus booster within 10 years
- anyone who has a large and/or dirty wound or burn who has not had a booster for more than 5 years

Cover all wounds with sterile or clean dressings, and attempt to keep the dressings clean and dry. When possible, apply a nonstick dressing (see chapter 5).

Inspect the wound every 24 to 48 hours for signs of infection (see following section). Change dressings every 24 to 48 hours or if they become wet and dirty.

After cleaning, insert sterile gauze into open wounds to hold the edges apart, then bandage.

WOUND INFECTION

All wounds can become infected. Deep dirty wounds, punctures, and bites have the highest risk of becoming infected. Dirt, gravel, and wood splinters left in a wound always produce infection. Animal and human bites also have a high risk of infection.

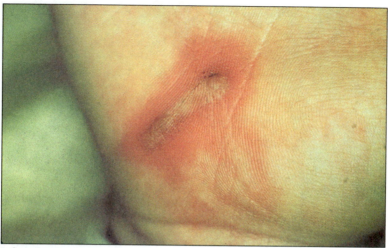

Infected wound

What to Look For

➤ redness spreading from the margins of the wound. As infection spreads away from the wound, the surrounding redness enlarges and one or more read streaks may appear leading from the wound toward the heart.

➤ warmth

➤ swelling

➤ increasing pain and tenderness

➤ pus, which will appear only if the wound is open and drains (It may be thick and creamy yellow or white, or thin and watery with a pink or light green color.)

➤ swollen, tender glands in the groin, armpit, or neck (whichever is closest to the infected wound)

➤ chills and fever, which indicate that an infection has spread into the blood and could become life threatening

➤ an abscess or boil, a collection of pus, may develop from a wound or in intact skin, starting as a pimple or small cyst (soft lump under the skin) and forming a white head (the natural drainage site)

What to Do

1. Clean the area.

2. Separate the wound edges gently to allow pus or infected fluids to escape.

3. Soak the wound in warm water or apply a warm wet compress (clean cloth dipped in bath-temperature water) for 15 minutes 4 times a day.

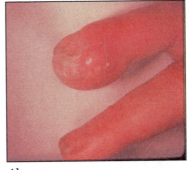

Abscess

4. Change the dressings as often as needed to keep them clean and dry.

5. Elevate the infected part.

6. Give aspirin, acetaminophen, or ibuprofen for pain.

7. Evacuate the victim if the infection does not resolve or becomes worse.

DRAINING AN ABCESS

ADVANCED PROCEDURE

To treat an abscess, release the pus. Wait until a natural drainage site, the white area in the center of the tender swelling, has developed. The formation of this central white head can be encouraged by frequent warm soaks or compresses. Try to open this "point" with the tip of a sharp knife blade, sterilized over a flame or in boiling water. The "point" has diminished feeling, but the surrounding skin is very sensitive. Make the incision rapidly. Numb the skin with ice, if available. Insert sterile gauze in the incision made by the knife blade, then bandage.

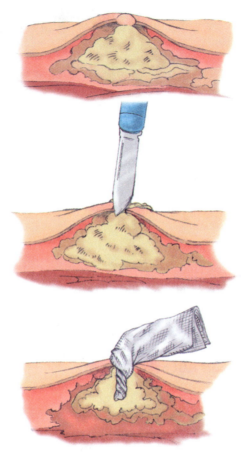

Treatment of an abscess: Make an incision in the central white head of the abscess. Insert a sterile gauze into the opening, then bandage.

SPECIAL WOUNDS

Amputations   Amputations are injuries in which parts of the body are completely cut off. Some amputated parts can be reattached surgically, so attempt to preserve the part.

What to Do (Amputations)

1. Check the ABCs.
2. Control bleeding.
3. Treat for shock.

If the amputated part can be found:

1. Rinse with clean water to remove dirt and debris. Do not scrub.
2. Wrap in sterile gauze or clean cloth.
3. Put in a plastic bag or waterproof container, then place on ice or snow in a second container.
4. Take the part to the hospital with the injured person.

Seek medical attention immediately. Amputated body parts unchilled for more than 6 hours have little chance of survival; 18 hours is the maximum survival time for a properly cooled part.

Fingertips amputated at the level of the nailbed or beyond cannot be reimplanted, but keep the tip, since it can be used as a skin graft. Skin and tissue lost through amputation at the end of a finger, not involving bone, will regrow and do not need reattachment. These injuries bleed for a long time; apply pressure and be patient.

 DO NOT

- **wrap the amputated part in a wet dressing or cloth; the tissues will become waterlogged, soft, and more difficult to reattach.**
- **bury the part in ice. Freezing results in unsuccessful reattachment.**
- **cut small skin "bridges," tendons, or other partial attachments. If the part is still attached, reposition it and wrap it firmly in a bulky, dry dressing.**

BLISTERS

A blister is a collection of fluid beneath the skin caused by excessive friction. (See appropriate sections for discussion of blisters from burns, frostbite, or contact with a poisonous plant.) To prevent blisters from forming, tape susceptible areas like the back of the heels with duct tape or adhesive tape, or cover with adhesive felt (moleskin) before blisters appear, especially if wearing new boots.

What to Do

1. Cover a "hot spot" or an unbroken blister with tape, duct tape, moleskin, or Spenco Second Skin™. Cover a larger area than the blister to avoid peeling of the dressing.

2. Use several layers of moleskin or molefoam (thicker than felt) cut in the shape of a doughnut that fits around the blister to relieve pressure.

 DO NOT

- use an adhesive strip bandage; friction will continue between the skin and the nonadherent pad.
- remove the tape until the hot spot or blister has healed.

Painful Unbroken Blisters   Clean with soap and water or disinfectant. Puncture several times around its edge with a needle sterilized over a flame. Gently press out the fluid. Do not remove the roof but cover it with a nonstick dressing, Spenco Second Skin™, or tape.

Broken Blisters   Clean surrounding skin with soap and water. Washing the broken surface is painful, but sand or dirt must be removed. Cover small blisters directly with tape. Cover large blisters with a nonstick pad, then apply tape or moleskin. It is often more comfortable to un-roof broken blisters (cut off the blister covering) and apply Spenco Second Skin™ directly to the wet surface. Unroof the blister if dirt or sand is seen under the skin and clean before applying dressing.

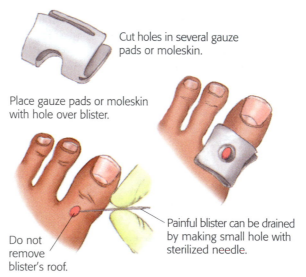

Cut holes in several gauze pads or moleskin.

Place gauze pads or moleskin with hole over blister.

Do not remove blister's roof.

Painful blister can be drained by making small hole with sterilized needle.

Blister care

Infected Blisters   Inspect painful blisters every 24 to 48 hours. Signs of infection include redness and tenderness extending beyond the edge of the blister, cloudy blister fluid, or pus. Cut away the dead skin overlying the blister and begin warm soaks.

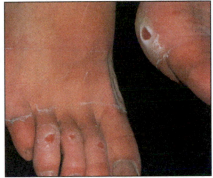

CLOSED WOUNDS— BRUISES

Blisters can be debilitating. Stop and tape over early hot spots before blisters like this form.

A bruise (contusion) is a collection of blood within or under the skin. Bleeding into deeper tissues can be extensive, especially in the thigh or buttock.

What to Look For

➤ pain and discoloration

➤ possible fracture; evaluate if the area is unusually painful, or moving the extremity is limited by pain (see chapter 8)

➤ blood appearing beneath the skin as a purple or yellow discoloration within a few hours or days after a superficial bruise

➤ over 5 to 10 days, a color change from purple/blue to yellow to green. The bruise spreads out under the skin, following gravity, to extend down the arm, leg, or face.

What to Do

1. Apply a cold pack, if available, for at least 20 minutes, 4 times a day, or longer for major bruises.

2. If a cold pack is not being applied, wrap firmly with an elastic bandage. Do not cut off circulation.

3. Evaluate travel needs. A few hours after a severe bruise in the leg or hip, the injured tissues may become so stiff and sore that the victim cannot walk comfortably. If it is necessary to walk to a trailhead or continue to a safe campsite, this may take precedence over immediate immobilization and cooling.

4. Seek medical attention for multiple bruises that appear spontaneously.

WOUNDS REQUIRING EVACUATION

Consider evacuation for

- uncontrolled or severe bleeding
- deep incisions, lacerations, or avulsions that
  - extend into muscle or bone
  - are located on or over a joint on the arm or leg
  - gape widely
  - contain a lot of dirt or debris
- severe hand or foot wounds
- large or deep puncture wounds
- large or deeply embedded objects
- bites, human and animal
- eyelid injuries with a break in the edge of the eyelid
- infected wounds
- amputations other than small areas of skin from fingertips

Most victims can walk and do not require helicopter or litter assistance for a wound.

Burns

Burns are caused by thermal, electrical, or radiant energy, and by certain chemicals. Although burns mainly involve the skin and underlying tissues, they can affect the eyes and respiratory passages. In the wilderness, the most common causes of burns are campfires, stoves, lightning, and sun.

The severity of a burn depends on its depth, extent, and location.

BURN CLASSIFICATION

Depth *First-degree (superficial) burns* affect the skin's outer layer (epidermis). The skin is mildly swollen, red, tender, and painful. Blisters do not form. *Second-degree (partial-thickness) burns* extend through the epidermis into the inner skin layer (dermis). There is moderate to severe pain, swelling, and blister formation. *Third-degree (full-thickness) burns* extend into the underlying fat and muscle. The skin is numb, looks charred, leathery, or pearly gray, and does not change color when pressed because it is dead.

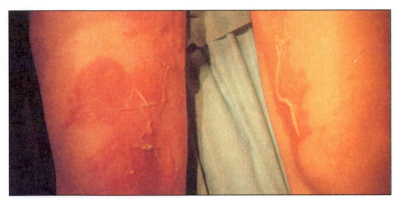

First- and second-degree burns

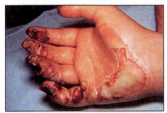

Second- and third-degree burns

A burn may contain all three degrees of damage: a third-degree burn in the center, surrounded by an area of second-degree burn with first-degree damage at the outermost edges.

Extent   Determine the extent of a burn by using the rule of 9s, which assigns a percentage of total skin surface to each part of the body. For small or scattered burns, estimate by using the palm of the victim's hand, which is approximately 1% of his or her body surface.

Location   Burns are serious if they

- involve the face, hands, feet, or genitals

- extend completely around the body or limb (circumferential burn), which may cause constriction of breathing or a tourniquet effect

- involve the respiratory tract, causing severe cough or shortness of breath; these burns will usually be associated with a burn of the face or mouth

- are associated with major injuries or illnesses

Severity   Burns are classified as *severe, moderate,* or *minor* depending on their location, extent, and depth. Burns that cover a large area are more severe than small, localized burns. Deep burns are more severe than those that are superficial. Painful burns are *not* as deep as painless burns, in which the nerve endings have been destroyed. Common sense will enable you to decide the severity of most burns.

Other Considerations   Particularly serious are major burns to children, the elderly, and those in poor health, and burns associated with other injuries.

Immediate Action   **Stop the burning!** Pour cold water onto the burned area immediately. If clothing is on fire and water is not available, tell the victim to roll on the ground, or wrap the person in a canvas tarp or wool jacket. Do not use polypropylene or nylon, which can melt and increase burn damage. Remove the victim from the flame or smoke-filled area. Cut off smoldering clothing immediately or soak it with water.

9%

9%

9%

9%

9%

1%

18% 18%

Rule of nines for calculating the extent of a burn. The entire head is 9%, each entire arm is 9% and each entire leg is 18%. The entire back is 18%.

What to Do at First

1. Check the ABCs, with special attention to the airway and breathing.

2. For small burns (less than 20% body surface), immerse in clean, cold water or cover with a cold, wet, clean cloth, snow, or ice pack for about 10 minutes to relieve pain. Cooling extensive burns (greater than 20% of body surface area) creates a risk of hypothermia.

3. Estimate depth and extent of burn and note any circumferential burns or critical area involvement.

4. Check for additional injuries, especially if the victim was in an explosion or under falling debris.

5. Remove jewelry and watches from burned extremities before swelling occurs. Remove belts and clothing from burned areas.

6. Keep burned skin clean and prevent blisters from breaking. (Burned skin has been sterilized by the heat.)

7. If the burn is second or third degree, cover with a dry, clean (preferably sterile) dressing. Cover a large burn with a clean sheet or blanket.

8. If the burn is on a hand or foot, put nonstick gauze pads between fingers or toes.

9. Evacuate the victim to medical care, unless the burn is minor in an otherwise healthy, uninjured adult. With moderate to severe burns, monitor airway and breathing at frequent intervals if there has been exposure to smoke or heat.

10. Encourage a large fluid intake in all victims except those with minimal burns.

11. Relieve pain and inflammation with aspirin or ibuprofen (acetaminophen relieves pain but not inflammation).

What to Do Later

First-Degree Burns

1. Apply a bland ointment or moisturizing cream (aloe vera) to soothe and keep skin soft.

2. Apply a dressing, which is not required but may reduce pain.

Second- and Third-Degree Burns

1. Wash burn gently with lukewarm water and mild soap. Avoid breaking blisters.

2. Apply a thin layer of antibiotic ointment (e.g., Bacitracin™).

3. Cover with nonstick dressing (preferably sterile but at least clean) held in place with a bandage.

4. If the burn is wet and oozing, remove dressing daily (you may have to soak off old dressings with clean, lukewarm water). Wash, reapply antibiotic ointment and a nonstick dressing.

Third-Degree Burns

1. Keep the area covered with a dry, sterile dressing or clean cloth.

ELECTRICAL BURNS

Electrical burns are rare in the wilderness but may occur from lightning strikes (chapter 15), in remote households, or job sites supplied with electric power. Sustained or high-voltage electricity produces entrance and exit skin burns. These can appear insignificant, but since the electric current penetrates deeply along the paths of least resistance (nerves and blood vessels), internal damage may be extensive. Respiratory and/or cardiac arrest may occur.

What to Do

1. Make sure the area is safe. Unplug, disconnect, or turn off the power. If this is impossible, call the power company for help (see chapter 15).

2. Check the ABCs. Be alert for possible fractures and/or head or spine injuries if the victim fell or was thrown to the ground by the shock. Treat unresponsiveness, respiratory arrest, and cardiac arrest (see chapter 9).

Electrical burn

3. Care for entrance and exit burn wounds.

4. Evacuate to medical care unless the victim recovers rapidly and completely, the burn is minimal, and injuries do not interfere with ability to travel.

SUNBURN

Sunburn is caused by ultraviolet rays in the UVB wavelength. Prolonged exposure to the sun is dangerous, especially in children, and increases the chances of skin cancer at a later age. The rays alter cells in the skin, causing cancer and premature aging. They also change pigments in the skin, increasing the amount of melanin (the golden tan). There is great variation in the tendency to become sunburned, but given enough exposure all skin will burn.

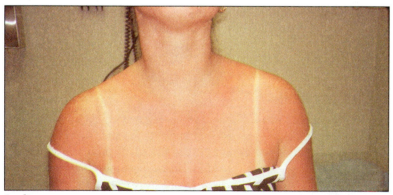

Sunburn

Sun reflects strongly off water, sand, and snow, and the effect is magnified by windburn. Ultraviolet rays penetrate hazy clouds, and while they are reduced by shadow, they are not eliminated. Preventing and reducing exposure of the skin is the cheapest, most effective way to avoid sunburn and to tan safely.

Clothing provides the best protection, but thin cotton clothes allow some rays to penetrate. Thicker, more opaque clothes can prevent exposure totally. Hats should have a wide brim both front and back. In environments with strong sun, long sleeves and pants are important.

Sun creams and lotions screen out the ultraviolet wavelengths that burn. The protective value of a sun screen is indicated by its SPF (sun protection factor) number. The higher the SPF number, the more the protection; 15 should be the minimum used by most people. Those with fair skin should use a screen with SPF 25–30.

Some screens contain para-aminobenzoic acid (PABA), an effective screen but one to which the wearer may be allergic. Alternative screens do not contain PABA. In extreme sun exposure an opaque screen such as zinc oxide can be used.

Sweating and swimming will quickly remove most screens. Waterproof screens are available and are preferable if the wearer is going to be in and out of water. Most screens should be reapplied every 2 to 4 hours.

What to Look For

➤ bright lobster-red skin color
➤ blisters

What to Do

1. Find shade if skin becomes pink and feels prickly and hot.

2. Soothe with cool compresses, baking soda compresses, or calamine lotion. Give antihistamine pills to decrease itching and ibuprofen to relieve the pain and inflammation.

3. Let burns heal. Most will do so in 2 to 3 days regardless of treatment.

CHAPTER 5

Dressings and Bandages

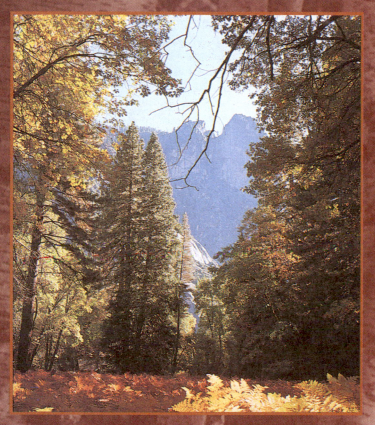

Dressings • Bandages • Applying and Removing a Dressing •
Bandaging Techniques

A dressing covers an open wound. Usually, you should use a sterile, commercially prepared dressing, but in the wilderness, you may have to improvise. A bandage holds the dressing in place. Also, use bandages to apply pressure over a dressing to control bleeding, prevent or reduce swelling, or provide support and stability for an injured joint or extremity.

Dressings

A dressing is used to control bleeding, keep the wound clean, prevent infection, absorb blood and wound drainage, and protect from further injury. Since the dressing covers an open wound, it should be sterile. If a commercial or other sterile dressing is not available, use clean cloth. The dressing should be larger than the wound; thick, soft, and compressible so that pressure is evenly distributed over the wound; absorbent (cotton is better than nylon or polyester); and lint-free so that fibers do not stick to the wound. Do not use cotton balls as dressing.

TYPES OF DRESSINGS

Use standard commercial dressings or improvise.

- **Gauze pads** are used for wounds requiring more than a small adhesive strip (e.g., a Band-Aid™). These are available in two common sizes (2-inch square; 4-inch square), sterile in separately wrapped packages of two, or nonsterile in bulk. Nonstick dressings (see below) are especially useful for burns or oozing wounds.

- **Adhesive strips** (e.g., Band-Aids™) come in many sizes and shapes. They can be improvised with a small piece of gauze and tape.

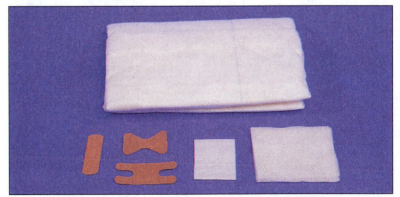

Dressing materials (front to back): adhesive strip, knuckle and fingertip bandages, nonstick Telfa™ pad, regular gauze pad, and trauma dressing

- **Trauma dressings** are large, thick, absorbent, and sterile. Sanitary napkins are an excellent substitute.

- **Nonstick dressings** have a plastic-like coating (Telfa™) or are impregnated with ointment (Adaptic™, Vaseline™, Xeroform™) to prevent adhering to wet wounds. To improvise, apply antibiotic ointment to the dressing or the wound.

- **Improvised dressings** can be any clean, absorbent, soft, and lint-free fabric. White cotton is optimal. Leaves, moss, and other natural products are *not* recommended. Paper sticks to wounds. If time allows, wash nonsterile cloth dressings in warm, soapy water and dry in the sun before using. To attempt sterilization, soak in bleach solution, boil, or carefully heat over a flame.

Bandages

A bandage is used with a dressing or to provide support for a joint or extremity injury. It should be clean, but it doesn't have to be sterile.

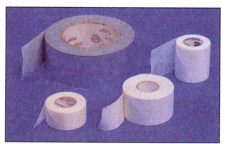

Several types of tape: paper tape, athletic tape, hypoallergenic tape, and duct tape

TYPES OF BANDAGES

- **Adhesive tape** includes white cloth "athletic" tape, which adheres even if wet. It can be used for taping sprains, blisters, and bandages, and can be split lengthwise down the middle for narrower sizes. Duct tape is an excellent substitute. Other types of medical tape that can be used for wound dressings include those that feel like "paper," "silk," and clear plastic (hypoallergenic).

- **Roller gauze bandages** are used to cover large wounds, to secure dressings, and to add extra layers. They come in various sizes (from 1 to 3 inches in width). Wider bandages can be folded as they are wrapped but are not as useful as "conforming" bandages.

- **Self-adhering, conforming bandages** are rolls of slightly elastic, gauzelike material. Two general styles are thin mesh or thicker, more absorbent mesh. The most useful widths for first aid kits are 2 and 4 inches. If there is room in the first aid kit for only one size, take the 3- or 4-inch width. Their self-adherent quality makes them

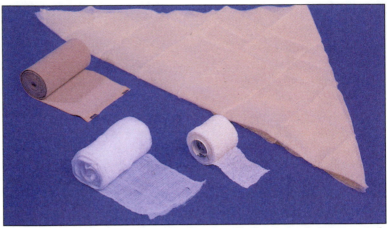

Bandage materials: gauze roller, self-adhering roller bandage, elastic wrap, and triangular bandage.

easy to use and they are easy to wrap around difficult areas such as joints.

- **Elastic (rubberized) bandages** are used for compression of sprains, strains, and contusions. They provide good protection for wounds. Do not wrap them too tightly.

- **Improvise** with a bandanna or strips of cotton cloth. Other sources of improvised bandages include socks, rolled t-shirts, belts, towels, and pillowcases.

- **Triangular bandages** can be used as slings or to tie splints or hold bandages. They are available commercially or can be made from a 36- to 40-inch square of material. A sling can be improvised using safety pins (see chapter 8).

Applying and Removing a Dressing

What to Do

1. Clean the wound (see page 62). Use gloves if there is any risk of blood contact (see page 60).

2. Use a dressing bigger than the wound. Hold the dressing by a corner. Lay the dressing directly onto the wound; do not slide it on.

3. Tape over the dressing or secure with a rolled bandage (see techniques below).

4. Fasten the bandage with
  * adhesive tape
  * safety pin(s)
  * clips provided with elastic bandage

5. Tie by either of these two methods:
  * **Loop method.** Simply tie the bandage ends that encircle the part from opposite directions. If necessary, reverse the direction of the bandage by looping it around a thumb or finger and continue back to the opposite side of the body part.
  * **Split-tail method.** Split the end of the bandage lengthwise for about 12 inches, and tie a knot to prevent further splitting. Pass the ends in opposite directions and tie. A square knot is preferred because it will not slip and can be easily untied. If the knot causes discomfort, pad under it.

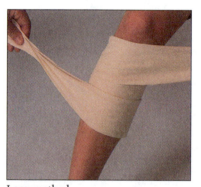
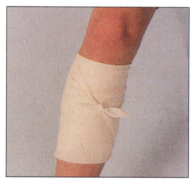

Loop method

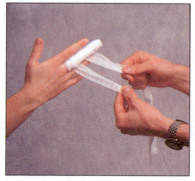
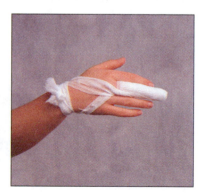

Split-tail method

A bulky wrap fashioned with a lot of turns will restrict most movement. If further immobilization is needed, add a splint or use a sling (see chapters 7 and 8).

 DO NOT

- touch the wound or the dressing that will be in contact with the wound.
- bandage tightly, restricting blood circulation.
- bandage so loosely that the dressing will slip. Bandages tend to stretch.
- cover fingers and toes unless they are injured. Leave some part visible to observe circulation.

Removing Dressings   If a dressing is stuck to a wound, soak it in warm water for 10 to 20 minutes, then gently peel off. Burn old dressings in a campfire.

Bandaging Techniques

BANDAGING THE EAR

If the bandage covers the ear, place strips of gauze or cloth behind the ear and the folds of the ear to maintain the normal anatomical position and shape of the ear.

BANDAGING THE HEAD

For a wound in the forehead or back of the scalp, wrap the head with a cloth cravat or a gauze roller bandage. To avoid bandaging over the ears, wrap low on the forehead and place ties under the bandage in front of the ears.

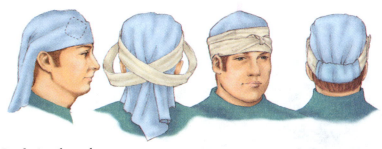

Bandaging the scalp

BANDAGING THE EXTREMITIES

To bandage an arm or a leg, begin at the narrow part of the limb and wrap toward the wider part of the extremity. Start with 2 anchor turns, then overlap the previous turn by ½ to ¾ of the width of the bandage. Tape or tie the end.

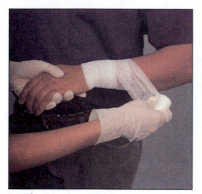 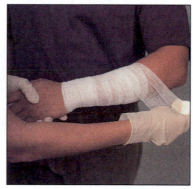

Bandaging extremities

BANDAGING THE ELBOW AND KNEE

After 2 anchor turns, wrap in a figure-8, making an **X** pattern across the joint.

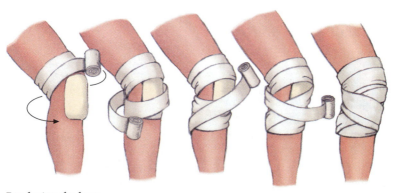

Bandaging the knee

BANDAGING THE WRIST AND HAND

Use a figure-8 wrap. Alternate encircling the wrist and hand, leaving the thumb free if uninjured.

A similar figure-8 technique works for dressing the fingers when a bulky wrap is needed to cover the entire digit or to limit movement. Wrapping around the wrist anchors the dressing so it does not slip off.

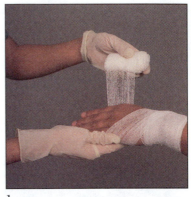

1.

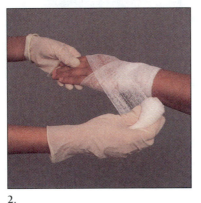

2.

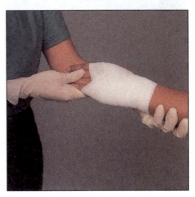

3.

Bandaging the wrist and hand

BANDAGING THE HAND

Place a dressing on the wound; place a roll or wad in the palm of the hand with the fingers curled around it. Wrap around the entire hand, anchoring and tying at the wrist. If the thumb and index finger are uninjured, they can be left out to maintain some use of the hand.

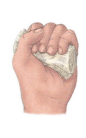
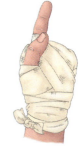

Bandaging the hand to prevent movement of the fingers

BANDAGING THE ANKLE AND FOOT

Use a figure-8 wrap. Alternate encircling the foot and ankle. The same technique is used for a dressing or compression wrap for an ankle sprain.

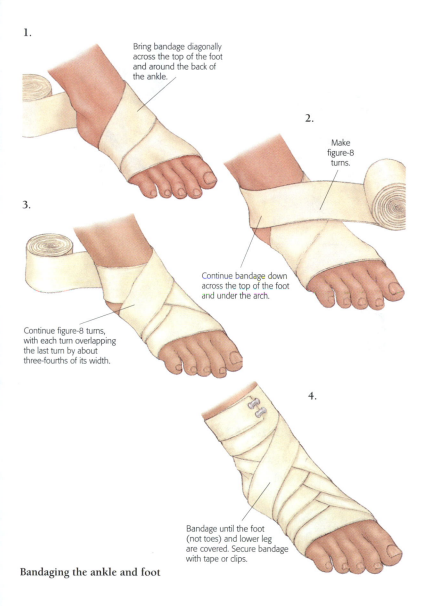

1.

Bring bandage diagonally across the top of the foot and around the back of the ankle.

2.

Make figure-8 turns.

3.

Continue bandage down across the top of the foot and under the arch.

Continue figure-8 turns, with each turn overlapping the last turn by about three-fourths of its width.

4.

Bandage until the foot (not toes) and lower leg are covered. Secure bandage with tape or clips.

Bandaging the ankle and foot

APPLYING A DRESSING OVER A WOUND WITHOUT PRESSURE

Use a doughnut to avoid pressure on a wound, for an open fracture or an embedded foreign body object, like glass or gravel, that cannot be removed.

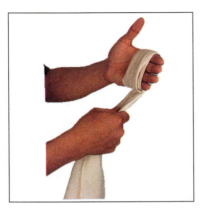
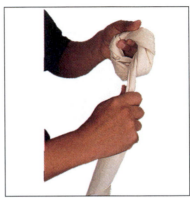

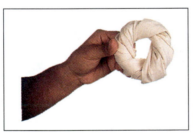

Making a "doughnut" to apply over a wound without pressure

SIGNS THAT A BANDAGE IS TOO TIGHT

- blue tinge of the fingernails or toenails
- blue or pale skin color and coldness of the extremity
- tingling or loss of sensation
- inability to move the fingers or toes
- pain beyond the bandage

CHAPTER 6

Head and Facial Injuries

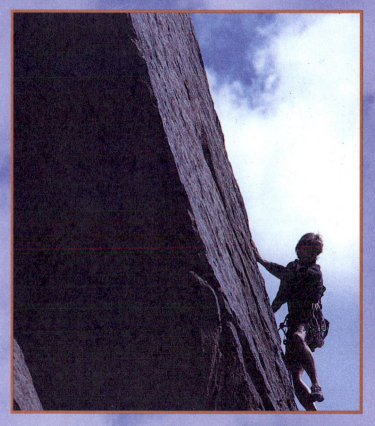

Scalp Wounds • Facial Wounds • Eyes • Ears • Nose • Throat • Jaw • Lips and Tongue • Dental Problems

Most people are afraid of being injured in the face or head. They fear the pain and possible disfigurement and automatically try to protect that area by raising an arm or turning away the head. Yet, injuries of the face and head are common. In a fall, the face or back of the head commonly strikes the ground. Severe injuries may damage the airway by breaking the nose or jaw and causing swelling inside the mouth. They may threaten eyesight, or may affect the brain, causing damage from a temporary concussion to permanent disability.

The possibility of injury to the brain and spinal cord must be considered in all facial and head injuries. In some instances the injury will be so superficial that it is obvious the spinal cord is intact and the brain undamaged. In others, there may be doubt about the integrity of the brain and spinal cord, instantly increasing the danger and complexity of management. The knowledge and ability to differentiate between these types of injury is, therefore, very important.

Scalp Wounds
What to Look For

➤ profuse bleeding because of the generous blood supply of the scalp. Extensive bleeding does not necessarily imply a brain or skull injury.

➤ blood pooled under the neck perhaps from an undetected scalp wound. Check the head, front, and back.

➤ shiny white bone, indicating a fracture

What to Do

1. Evaluate for head and spinal injury (see page 141).

2. Control bleeding with pressure.

3. When bleeding has been controlled, remove dirt, blood clots, and hair from the wound; then wash with soap and water. Cover the wound with a sterile compress.

4. Twist small bundles of hair and tie them across the wound, drawing the edges snugly together. Make sure there is no dirt or debris in the wound before it is closed.

5. If oozing continues, do not remove the first blood-soaked dressing, but add another dressing over it.

6. Monitor the victim for brain injury using the AVPU scale (see page 47).

7. Evacuate the victim if
 • the laceration is extensive
 • infection is likely because of wound contamination
 • there is significant involvement of the face
 • the injury is associated with signs of brain injury

Facial Wounds
What to Look For

➤ extensive bleeding. May be superficial or involve the cavity of the mouth, the eyelids, or the ears.

What to Do

1. Clean the wound with soap and water.

2. If the wound is large, restore the skin flaps as best as you can and apply a dressing.

3. Evacuate all but trivial injuries. Helicopter evacuation is not necessary for a simple laceration; wounds may be safely closed several days later.

FACIAL FRACTURE

The bony ring around the eye socket may be broken and deformed.

What to Look For

➤ eyeball sunk inward, causing double vision

➤ cheek on one side is tender and flatter than on the other side

➤ a step in the smooth lower rim of the orbit

➤ pain on chewing or opening the mouth widely

What to Do

1. Patch one eye to correct double vision.

2. Evacuate to a surgeon.

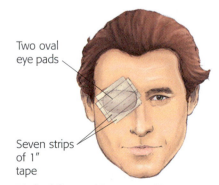

Two oval eye pads

Seven strips of 1" tape

Method for patching an eye. Use a double eye patch held in place with seven strips of 1" tape.

Eyes

Most first aiders are nervous about examining the eye closely. However, careful observation is essential for an accurate assessment. If your camera has a detachable lens, look for foreign objects by using the camera lens as a magnifier. Remove the lens from the camera and reverse it so that the end attached to the camera now faces the eye.

What to Do

1. Test the vision in each eye separately, covering one eye at a time. Ask the victim to read normal print, or, if unable, to count fingers.
2. Covering one eye at a time, ask the victim to look straight at the bridge of your nose. Ask if there are any blind spots or dark areas in the vision.

INFECTION

Though not an injury, this is a common eye problem in the wilderness. The eye becomes red and itchy ("pinkeye").

What to Look For

➤ red eye

➤ lids stuck together with pus, especially in the morning after waking up

What to Do

1. Wash the eye frequently with warm water.
2. Apply antibiotic eye drops or antibiotic eye ointment (see appendix B) in *both* eyes 3 to 4 times a day.
3. Avoid spreading infection to other people. Wash hands and don't share towels.

NONPENETRATING INJURY

Subconjunctival hemorrhage can occur after a mild blow to the eye, after rubbing the eye during sleep, or after sneezing or vomiting. No treatment is necessary.

What to Look For

➤ blood under the white of the eye but no change in vision. The bright red blood looks, but is not, dangerous.

FOREIGN BODY

A speck of dirt, fire ash, or metal may become embedded in the cornea or lodged under either of the lids. This is *very* uncomfortable.

What to Look For

➤ Inspect the cornea with magnification.

➤ Look under both lids. Pull down the lower lid; turn the upper lid over a match stick.

What to Do

1. Wash the eye with water; reexamine and wash again if foreign body still present, or

2. Carefully remove the speck with a folded corner of a damp gauze, cloth, or cotton tip.

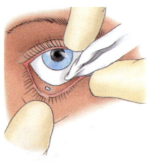

a. If tears or gentle flushing do not remove object, gently pull lower lid down. Remove an object by gently flushing with lukewarm water or a wet sterile gauze.

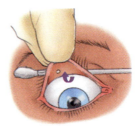

c. Fold the lid over the swab or matchstick. Remove an object by gently flushing with lukewarm water or a wet sterile gauze.

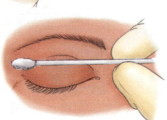

b. Tell the person to look down. Pull gently downward on upper eyelashes. Lay a swab or match stick across the top of the lid.

Removing foreign object from the eye

SCRATCH

A twig, pine needle, or flying wood chip may scratch the eyeball. The painful scratchy feeling usually heals in 24 to 48 hours.

What to Look For

➤ tearing, blurred vision, pain

What to Do

1. If available, use tannic acid by dropping cold tea from a used teabag into the eye every hour.
2. Do not patch or pad the eye; dark glasses are sufficient.
3. Give painkillers. If pain persists, consider an infection (pus in eye), an ulcer (visible), or inflammation (blurred vision). The victim may need medical care.

ULTRAVIOLET BURN ("SNOWBLINDNESS")

Sun reflecting strongly off snow and light-colored rocks can burn the cornea, causing intense pain.

What to Look For

➤ redness, tearing, light sensitivity, slight clouding of the cornea soon after exposure

➤ swelling of the conjunctiva, which closes the eyes tightly, leading to temporary "blindness"

➤ blistering of the cornea, which blurs vision

To prevent snowblindness, wear dark glasses or goggles. In an emergency cut horizontal slits or punch multiple pinholes in a piece of cardboard or duct tape doubled on itself, and tie it around the head with string. Cut side shields to prevent glare.

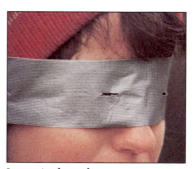

Improvised goggles

What to Do

1. Give painkillers and drip cold tea (tannic acid) into the eye frequently.
2. Lead or carry the victim to safety.
3. After reaching safety, treat both eyes as if they have suffered a severe corneal scratch (see above). The pain and swelling should subside in a day.

CHEMICAL BURNS (BATTERY ACID, LIME, ETC.)

Acid burns usually heal quickly, like an abrasion or ultraviolet burn; alkali burns are severe and need urgent medical care.

What to Do

1. Find out what entered the eye. Was it acid or alkali?

2. Irrigate the eye with water immediately, continuously, and gently for 20 minutes. Remove any chemical particles.

BRUISING

A black eye in itself is usually not serious, as the bony rim of the eye socket—not the eye—is bruised.

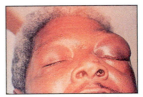

Swelling of eyelid due to blow to eye

What to Look For

➤ decreased vision (you may need to hold the eye open to evaluate if lids are swollen shut)

➤ blood filling the front of the eye. After a few hours the blood settles by gravity; a level of blood can be seen in the front of the eye, and vision clears.

➤ increasing pain, redness, tearing, and light sensitivity 1 to 3 days after a blow to the eye (indicating inflammation inside the eye or iris)

What to Do

1. Apply a cold pack for about 15 minutes. Do not press on the eye.

2. Evacuate the victim speedily if there is any alteration in vision, or blood in the eye or iris.

FROZEN EYELASHES

During a blizzard, eyelashes may become frozen together so that the eye cannot be opened. Warm the eye with a hand to melt the ice. No harm will come to the eye.

OPEN INJURY (PENETRATING)

An open injury is caused by a high-velocity metal fragment such as from a hammer striking a metal or an axe striking rock. Often the wound in the cornea is tiny and seals over, disguising the injury.

What to Look For

➤ red, painful eye with tearing and light sensitivity

➤ pear-shaped pupil

➤ impaired vision

What to Do

1. Protect the eye with a cardboard shield or a doughnut-shaped rolled bandage (depends upon the length of the penetrating object).

2. Administer painkillers.

3. Evacuate to an eye surgeon immediately.

PENETRATING INJURY

Objects may become caught in the eyeball. Do not push the object further into the eye by applying a patch. Evacuate the victim as soon as possible.

Protect the injured eye with a paper cup, cardboard folded into a cone, or doughnut-shaped pad made from roller gauze bandage or cravat bandage.

EYELID INJURY

If an eyelid is infected or lacerated, always check the globe of the eye for associated injury.

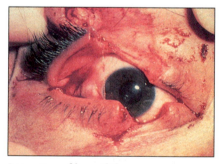

Laceration of lower lid

What to Look For

➤ a cut in the lid margin creating a notch

➤ a cut in the corner of the eye near the nose where the tear ducts lie

What to Do

1. Evacuate the victim to a surgeon.

LOST EYEGLASSES

All eyeglass wearers should take an extra pair of glasses on a wilderness trip. A cheap pair of drugstore glasses may be sufficient to allow the wearer to function adequately. Nearsighted people can increase the acuity of their vision by looking through cardboard or duct tape goggles punched with multiple pinholes.

Ears

Generally, ear problems do not threaten a person's life. But in the wilderness, small round objects or insects may lodge in the ear canal and damage hearing if not treated.

What to Do

1. Pull the earlobe upward and backward to straighten the canal. Lubricate with vegetable or mineral oil. Turn the head on one side and shake vigorously.

2. Flush the ear with clean, warm water using a syringe. Use moderate pressure but do not block the ear canal with the syringe. Vegetable objects, such as beans, may swell in contact with water; try an oil lubricant (not motor oil) first.

3. Insects are best removed by first drowning them with a drop of mineral or vegetable cooking oil. If the insect can be seen, remove it carefully with tweezers; otherwise flush.

4. Remove visible foreign bodies from the canal with tweezers.

 DO NOT
- **probe with matchsticks or twigs; this may damage the eardrum.**

Nose
NOSEBLEED

Bleeding usually stops on its own after a few minutes with pressure alone. On rare occasions an uncontrollable nosebleed may threaten the victim's life. Bleeding typically comes from a spot that cannot be seen on the center divider (septum).

What to Look For

➤ bleeding from one or both nostrils

What to Do

1. Have the victim lean slightly forward, head bowed.

2. Squeeze the nose against the bones for 5 minutes.

3. If bleeding continues, blow the nose gently or sniff to remove clots. If available, spray nose 4 times on both sides with nasal decongestant spray (e.g., Afrin™, Neo-Synephrin™).

4. If bleeding continues, squeeze the nose again for 5 minutes.

5. Place a cold compress, preferably of ice or snow wrapped in a damp cloth, across the bridge of the nose.

6. Encourage breathing through the mouth.

7. Avoid picking at clots, rubbing, or blowing the nose.

BROKEN NOSE

What to Look For

➤ swollen, tender, and possibly misshapen nose

➤ bleeding and difficulty in breathing through the nostril

➤ black eyes, which usually appear 1 to 2 days after the nose has been broken. Check for eye injury by testing vision of both eyes.

What to Do

1. Apply ice or a cold pack to reduce the swelling and bleeding. Treat a nosebleed as described above.

A nasal fracture and two black eyes may look bad, but, without deformity, need no treatment. Even with some deformity this is not an urgent problem. A surgeon can deal with a deformed fracture a week later.

 DO NOT

• try to straighten a crooked nose.

Throat
SWALLOWED FOREIGN BODY

A small bone or piece of food can become stuck in the throat or esophagus. Objects stuck in the throat require immediate action.

What to Look For

➤ Meat or food stuck in the esophagus is painful and may cause vomiting, but the victim can breathe and speak normally.

➤ A piece of meat or other food stuck in the throat or at the vocal cords causes choking and the victim cannot speak or breathe.

What to Do

1. For obstructed breathing, use abdominal thrusts (Heimlich maneuver) (see appendix A).

2. For food stuck in the esophagus, have the victim sip liquids to try and wash the piece down. It may be possible to regurgitate the food, but this can take several hours. Try to see a small bone in the throat by pushing the tongue down with the handle of a spoon. Bones commonly lodge at the base of the tongue or around the edge of the tonsil. If you can see the bone, grasp it with tweezers or rub it off with a cotton tip. If not seen, have victim swallow dry bread to dislodge it.

Jaw
FRACTURE
What to Look For

➤ injury to jaw or face

➤ inability to chew or clench the teeth; jaws do not close accurately

➤ pain and tenderness along the jawbone (feel along the lower and inner edge to avoid simple bruises) or at the joint in front of the ear (there are often two areas of fracture)

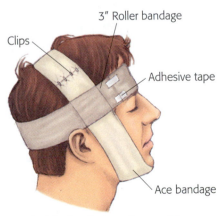

Method for bandaging a fractured jaw

> signs that may indicate other facial bone fractures include double vision, a flattened cheek, or numbness on one side of the nose and lip

What to Do

1. Guide the lower jaw into position against the upper jaw and secure with a cravat bandage tied around the head and under the jaw. *Be sure the cravat bandage can be removed rapidly should the victim vomit!*

2. Feed a fluid diet until the jaw can be seen by a dentist or oral surgeon.

DISLOCATION

What to Look For

> no injury, but a history of the jaw popping out with a yawn or wide opening of the mouth

> inability of jaw to close

> misalignment

> pain in front of the ears (temporomandibular joint, or TMJ) but no tenderness in lower arch of jaw

Joint socket in skull   Top of jaw

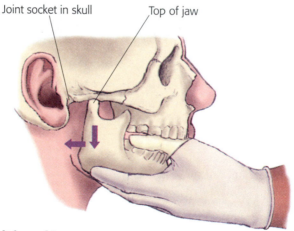

Fixing a dislocated jaw

What to Do

1. Support the lower jaw with the fingers of both hands, place your thumbs over the person's molars (padded to prevent biting), then push steadily down and backward. The jaw should slide back into place.

2. Secure with a cravat for a few days and feed liquids.

Lips and Tongue

The tongue and lips are usually cut by the teeth. Bleeding is the major problem due to a rich blood supply. The laceration may be on one side or all the way through, in the middle or at the edge.

What to Do

1. Control bleeding by direct pressure with a gauze or cloth, pinched with the fingers.

2. Apply ice, if available.

3. Soak gauze or cloth with nasal decongestant spray or drops (e.g., Afrin™ or Neo-Synephrin™), then apply to wound.

4. Avoid crumbly foods.

5. Rinse well after eating.

Evacuate in the event of

- full-thickness lacerations of the tongue, longer than ½ inch
- significant-sized flaps of the lips or the edge of the tongue that do not stay in place
- cuts of the lip that extend through the junction of the lip and facial skin wounds that extend through the lips

Dental Problems
TOOTHACHE

Prevent toothache with a careful dental check, especially before a long trip or expedition. Clean teeth regularly. If there is no toothbrush, rub the teeth with salt or a peeled green stick. Chewing sugarless gum cleans the mouth and gums.

CAVITIES

A cavity due to decay, a lost filling, or a fractured tooth lays bare the sensitive dentin under the enamel.

What to Look For

➤ sensitivity to heat, cold, or sweets; dental pain may ache, throb, or sear and be difficult to localize to a particular tooth. It often affects adjacent teeth and may spread from the upper jaw to the lower and vice versa, but never across the midline.

➤ sensitivity to touch: tap the teeth gently, with something metal (e.g., spoon handle), on the top and side. A diseased tooth will hurt.

What to Do

1. Rinse and flush the mouth.

2. Apply oil of cloves on a Q-tip to the cavity.

3. Apply temporary dressing of synthetic tooth cement (Cavit™). Push the dressing paste into the cavity with a finger and press it down with a matchstick. Have the person bite it into place before it sets.

ABSCESS

What to Look For

➤ swelling of the gums around the diseased tooth

➤ swelling of the jaw visible in the face

➤ foul breath

➤ pain, exacerbated by tapping the tooth

What to Do

1. Rinse the mouth with warm water to soothe, cleanse, and encourage pus to discharge into the mouth.

2. Give aspirin or ibuprofen for pain. If the person has antibiotics, the best choices for antibiotics are amoxicillin or erythromycin, 500 mg 4 times a day; the next best choice is penicillin. See appendix B for use of antibiotics.

3. See a dentist after leaving the wilderness.

DO NOT
- pull the tooth out.
- probe with a needle.

AVULSED (KNOCKED-OUT) TOOTH

What to Do

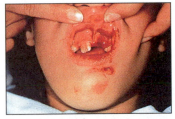

Tooth knocked from upper jaw

1. Give the victim a warm salt mouthwash.

2. Rinse the tooth gently in clean water and replace it immediately in the socket. Hold it in place with pressure by clenching teeth together. Otherwise, transport by keeping the tooth between the cheek and gums.

3. Evacuate the victim to a dentist as soon as possible.

CHAPTER 7

Bone, Joint, and Muscle Injuries

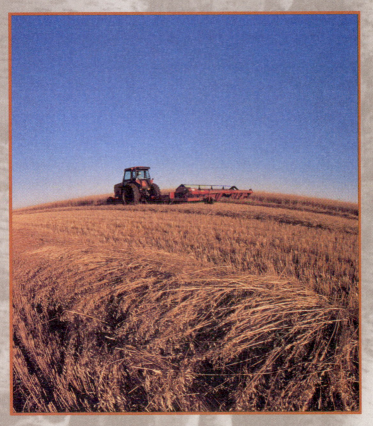

Bone Injuries • Joint Injuries • Muscle Injuries

Sprains, strains, contusions, fractures, and dislocations of the extremities are among the most common injuries in the wilderness. The treatment of these injuries depends on the expertise of those in the party and the distance from medical help.

Managing these injuries requires common sense, some diagnostic skills, and sensitivity to the needs of the victim and the group. For example, with a painful ankle injury, consider the desire and ability of the person to walk, whether people are available for transportation, the terrain, weather, and distance involved. Try to encourage self-rescue without calling for outside help. Support the ankle with a splint or tape and use an ice axe, ski pole, or wooden stick for balance. Although the decision to walk may cause more pain, this might be safer than waiting for help.

A *fracture* is a break or crack in a bone. Important distinctions are whether a fracture is deformed or not and whether it is closed or open. In a closed fracture, the skin has no wound near the fracture site. In an open fracture, the skin overlying the fracture is broken by bone protruding through the skin or by the blow that produced the fracture (see page 116 for management).

A *dislocation* occurs when the bone-ends at a joint are separated and out of alignment, creating a deformity. A *strain* is a tearing injury of muscle. It occurs when muscle is stretched beyond its normal limit

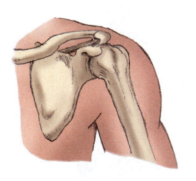
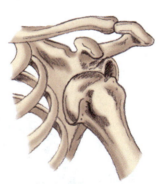

Normal position   Dislocated

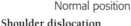

Shoulder dislocation

or is stretched suddenly and forcibly. A *sprain* occurs when a ligament (the tough tissue that holds bones together) is stretched beyond its limit, causing a minor pull or major tear.

Contusions (bruises) result from a blow to skin, muscle, or other soft tissues overlying bones. There is bleeding into the surrounding tissues.

Muscle cramps are uncontrolled muscle spasms.

Bone Injuries
ASSESSMENT

It may be difficult to tell if a bone is fractured. Signs and symptoms of a fracture may include deformity, an open wound, tenderness, and swelling. Dislocations, severe strains, sprains, and even contusions may cause swelling and pain that mimic fractures. When in doubt, treat the injury as a fracture. Use the sequence "ask, look, and feel" to examine an extremity.

Ask how the injury occurred. What was the mechanism of injury? (Severe impact accidents or falls are more likely to cause a fracture.) Where does it hurt? How severe is the pain? Can you use the injured part? A snapping sound can be heard with fractures and with ligament or muscle tears (sprains and strains).

Look at the injury for deformity, open wounds, and swelling.

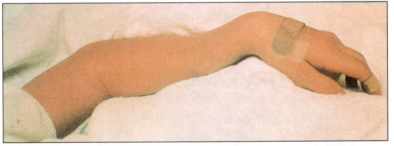

Deformed forearm fracture demonstrating angulation

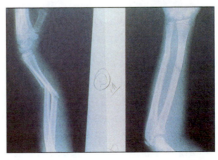

- Deformity is not always obvious. Compare the injured side to the uninjured side. Severe deformity (angulation), shortening, or rotation of the extremity when compared with the opposite extremity indicates a bone injury.

- Open wound (e.g., puncture or laceration) overlying an obvious deformity or unstable bone is considered an open fracture. Bone is not always seen in the wound. Persistent oozing of blood despite pressure on the skin wound is another clue to an open fracture. An abrasion or a clearly superficial cut does not imply an open fracture.

PEDIATRIC NOTE   Children's bones are more elastic but not as strong as adults' because they are still growing. In adults a fracture is usually a complete break in the continuity of a bone. A child's fracture, however, may be incomplete: a "greenstick" partial fracture, a gentle but distinct bending of the bone called plastic deformity, or a buckling of the bone. The ligaments that join bones together at joints are relatively stronger than the bones they connect, and in some injuries segments of bone may be pulled away, attached to a ligament that remains untorn. Therefore, a child should be presumed to have a fracture rather than a sprain if there is localized pain and swelling near a joint.

- Swelling and bruising caused by bleeding from the bone or overlying muscle damage occur rapidly after a fracture. Swelling and bruising also occur with contusions and strains.

- Loss of use where pain and muscle spasm restrict movement of nearby joints. Ask the victim to move the injured limb. Support the injured area and gently move the involved joints for the victim. If this causes severe pain or grating/cracking (crepitus), a fracture is likely. Grating with no history of injury may indicate tendonitis.

Feel for tenderness and the grating sensation of broken-bone movement.

- Tenderness and pain are found at the site of injury. Feel gently along the bone; a fracture will be tender when felt from either side of the bone, whereas a bruise will be tender only on the side of impact.

- Abnormal movement is associated with crunching sounds or grating sensations (crepitus) and causes severe pain.

TREATMENT
What to Do

1. Control bleeding. Treat the victim for shock if present (see pages 149–151).

2. Expose the injury. Gently remove clothing covering the injured area. Cut clothing at the seams if necessary to avoid excessive movement and pain. In cold environments, remove as little clothing as possible to examine the person.

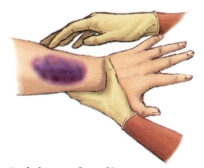

Feel along surface of bone opposite from bruise and swelling. If no tenderness, fracture is unlikely.

3. Check damage to blood vessels and nerves. A serious complication of a fracture is decreased blood flow (circulation) to the extremity. Major blood vessels lie close to bone, so a fracture or dislocation that causes a marked deformity of the bone may stretch, compress or pinch adjacent blood vessels and nerves. Rarely are vessels or nerves actually torn by bone fragments.

   * *Check circulation.* Without blood, the tissues of the arms and legs cannot survive for more than 2 or 3 hours. Deformity and swelling can reduce the blood flow significantly, but circulation is rarely blocked or disrupted completely. Numbness and bluish color indicate decreased circulation. Splinting or wrapping too tightly can also obstruct blood flow.

     Compare the color of the hand or foot on the injured and uninjured sides. A blue or pale limb beyond an injury may indicate diminished circulation. Press on the tip of a nail or the pad of a finger or toe to blanch the skin. The pink color should return as quickly on the injured as on the uninjured side. Check the pulse at the wrist or the ankle. Feel the uninjured side first to locate the pulse. Swelling over the area will make the pulse difficult or impossible to feel. If the pulse is felt, mark the spot with a pen so it can be found again.

   * *Assess sensation.* Major nerves also lie close to bone and can be torn, bruised, stretched, or pinched by adjacent broken bone. The part may be numb but with normal circulation. This is not an urgent problem unless associated with impaired circulation.

Ask whether the hand or foot has normal sensation. Evaluate numbness carefully; pain and hyperventilation (excessively deep breathing) can produce numbness. Ask if squeezing can be felt on exposed toes and fingers. Touch with something sharp (safety pin or pine needle). Inability to detect a pinprick is a sign of nerve or spinal cord damage or an early sign of restricted blood supply.

- *Assess movement.* If the victim can wiggle the toes or fingers, the nerves to the muscles are working. Pain may restrict movement, but not completely.

4. Realign deformities. Correct angles and deformities of the bones when injuries occur where evacuation will require many hours or days. Straighten bones immediately to restore circulation that is impaired from a fracture or dislocation. This differs from first aid in urban areas, where you "splint it as it lies."

5. Splint the fracture to stabilize it. Most broken bones are not displaced and can be stabilized in the position in which they are found. Sprains and strains also need support. Stabilize all fractures and dislocations before moving the victim. When in doubt, apply a splint.

How to Apply Traction to Deformed Fractures

1. Explain to the victim that straightening the fracture may cause pain, but the pain will decrease when the fracture is straightened and splinted.

2. Grasp an injured arm firmly with both hands—one hand above the injury site and the other below it. Increase the pull gradually to exert steady, firm traction along the long axis of the bone. Pull an injured leg with both hands while the victim's body acts as an anchor or another person holds the upper leg in place. Compare the injured side with the normal side to see what the straightened extremity should look like. Traction may not pull the limb back into perfect alignment, but that can be achieved later in the hospital. Techniques for reducing specific fractures and dislocations are discussed in chapter 8.

3. Stop pulling if the victim feels intolerable pain or if several minutes of traction fail to improve the position.

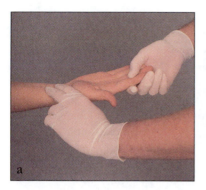
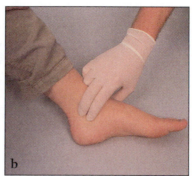
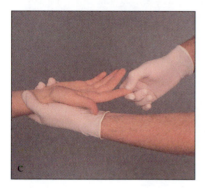
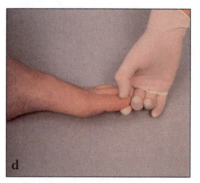
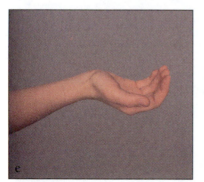
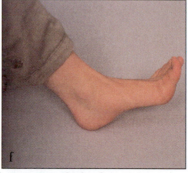

Checking extremities   a. Radial pulse   b. Posterior tibial pulse   c. Sensation: squeeze one or more toes.   d. Circulation: Check color return after pressure on nail or tip.   e, f. Movement: Have the victim wiggle fingers or toes. Movement may be decreased due to pain. Note: Gloves are not necessary unless there is bloody injury.

- Have another person apply gentle traction until you can apply a splint.
- By preventing movement, a splint will minimize pain; prevent further damage to muscle, nerves, and blood vessels; prevent a closed fracture from becoming an open fracture; reduce bleeding and swelling; facilitate travel or evacuation.

For maximum immobilization, stabilize the joint above and below the injury. For example, a fractured forearm requires a splint long enough to secure the wrist and the elbow. If you stabilize the wrist only, the forearm bone (radius) can still move whenever the elbow turns. If the injury is near a joint, splinting only that joint may provide adequate comfort while allowing better function. For an injured joint, stabilize the bone above and below. For example, for a knee injury, secure the splint at both the thigh and lower leg. Balance adequate immobilization

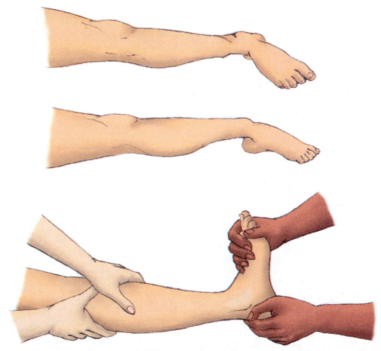

Correct major angulation and deformities by applying traction along normal axis of the bone. The goal is to improve alignment, not to achieve optimal position for healing (reduction).

with the need for comfort and function. Place splint materials on both sides of the injured part ("sandwich splint") to prevent the part from turning or twisting.

You may have to improvise splints with clothing, foam sleeping pads, backpack stays, pillows, branches, or ski poles. Splints should be padded for comfort and rigid for safety. The victim will tell you if the splint works. Monitor circulation and sensation before and after applying the splint, and periodically while the splint is in place, to ensure that it is not too tight. Ask the victim to tell you if pain or sensation changes.

Techniques of splinting are described under the individual injuries.

6. Limit swelling and pain with RICE (see below).

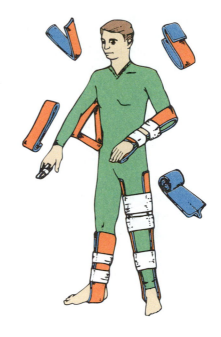

SAM™ splint, a good splint to carry in your first aid kit, is made of a malleable sheet of aluminum sandwiched between foam padding. It weighs very little and can be rolled or folded flat to carry. It can be molded to any part of the body. Forming a longitudinal fold or groove in the splint adds strength.

The acronym **RICE** is used to remember first aid procedures for contusions (bruises), strains, sprains, dislocations, and fractures.

R: Rest. Stop or decrease use of the injured part with the aid of splints, wraps, slings, and periods of rest.

I: Ice. Apply an ice pack frequently during the first 48 hours. In the wilderness, use snow or cold water if ice is unavailable. Skin treated with cold passes through four states: cold, burning, aching, and numbness. When it becomes numb (in about 20 minutes), remove the ice pack. Cold constricts the blood vessels in the injured area, which reduces swelling, dulls pain, and relieves muscle spasm. The sooner cold is applied, the better. To intensify the cold, place a wet cloth between the skin and ice pack.

C: Compression. Compression of the injured area may limit internal bleeding around the injury. Less bleeding or bruising means less soreness and limitation of movement and a faster recovery time, especially for muscle or ligament injuries. Apply cold about every 2 to 3 hours; maintain compression at other times. At night, loosen but do not remove the elastic bandage.

- Use an elastic bandage or wrap snugly with strips of cloth.

- Start the elastic bandage several inches below the injury or at the base of the fingers or toes and wrap in an upward, overlapping spiral, starting with even and somewhat tight pressure, then gradually wrapping looser above the injury.

- **Do NOT** apply an elastic bandage too tightly; they can restrict circulation. Stretch the elastic bandage to about half its maximum length for adequate compression.

- Leave fingers and toes exposed to see color changes. Compare the color and movement of the toes or fingers of the injured extremity with the uninjured extremity.

- If there is pale skin, numbness, or tingling, remove the elastic bandage and rewrap the area less tightly.

E: Elevation. Elevating the injured limb helps limit bleeding and minimizes swelling.

OPEN FRACTURES

What to Do

1. Clean off dirt and debris and irrigate the bone-end (see chapter 4).

2. Do not push the bone-end back under the skin. Gently try to correct deformities, as described above. This will usually return the bone-end below the skin.

3. Cover all open fracture wounds with a dry, sterile dressing before applying a splint.

4. Make a written note of how much bone is protruding and if there is debris on the bone or in the wound before immediate evacuation to an orthopedic surgeon.

5. Splint and wrap the extremity.

Joint Injuries
DISLOCATIONS

A dislocation occurs when a joint comes apart and stays apart with the bone-ends no longer in their usual position. The main sign of a dislocation is deformity—often a bizarre appearance compared to the uninjured side. Dislocations have signs and symptoms similar to those of a fracture: deformity, severe pain, and the inability of the victim to move the injured joint. The shoulders, elbows, fingers, hips, kneecaps, and ankles are the joints most frequently affected.

What to Do

1. Evaluation and management of dislocations are similar to those of fractures. If medical care will be delayed or there is compromised circulation, attempt to reduce (put back in place) the dislocation of the shoulder, finger, or kneecap.

SPRAINS

A sprain is an injury to a joint in which the ligaments and other tissues are damaged by stretching or twisting. The ankles, knees, and thumbs are the joints most often sprained. The main symptoms include swelling, pain, decreased movement, and limited use of the joint. Bruising appears within hours to days. It often is difficult to distinguish between a severe sprain and a fracture. Some sprains involve small fractures, but this does not change the management in the field.

What to Do

1. Evaluate as for a fracture.
2. Apply RICE procedures.
3. Splint or tape for support (see specific injuries in chapter 8).

Muscle Injuries
STRAINS

A muscle strain, also known as a muscle pull, occurs when a muscle is stretched beyond its normal range of motion, tearing some of the fibers.

What to Look For

➤ limited movement due to pain and stiffness

➤ variable tenderness

➤ variable swelling and bruising depending on the extent of damage

➤ delayed symptoms, possibly for 1 to 2 days depending on the severity of injury

What to Do

1. Apply RICE procedures.
2. Stretch gently.

MUSCLE CRAMPS

A cramp is an uncontrolled spasm and contraction resulting in sudden pain and restriction of movement.

What to Do

Try one or more of the following:

- Have the victim gently stretch the affected muscle.
- Apply steady pressure over the muscle
- Apply ice to the cramped muscle.
- If the cramping has followed hard exertion in the heat, give mildly salted water (¼ to 1 level teaspoon in 1 quart of water) or a commercial electrolyte drink.
- For nocturnal cramps, try taking diphenhydramine (Benadryl™) at bedtime.

CHAPTER 8

Specific Bone and Joint Injuries

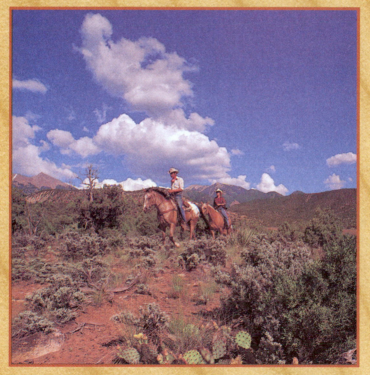

Upper Extremities • Lower Extremities • Spine •

Moving a Victim with a Spinal Injury •

When to Remove Spinal Immobilization •

Guidelines for Evacuation of Musculoskeletal Injuries

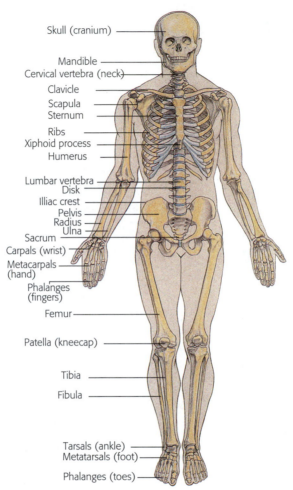

Skull (cranium)

Mandible
Cervical vertebra (neck)
Clavicle
Scapula
Sternum
Ribs
Xiphoid process
Humerus
Lumbar vertebra
Disk
Illiac crest
Pelvis
Radius
Ulna
Sacrum
Carpals (wrist)
Metacarpals
(hand)
Phalanges
(fingers)
Femur

Patella (kneecap)

Tibia

Fibula

Tarsals (ankle)
Metatarsals (foot)
Phalanges (toes)

The skeletal system

Managing specific bone and joint injuries in remote environments requires common sense, some diagnostic skills, and sensitivity to the needs of the victim and the group. For example, with a painful ankle injury, consider the desire and ability of the person to walk; whether people are available for transportation; and the terrain, weather, and distance involved. Try to encourage self-rescue without calling for outside help. Support the ankle with a splint or tape and use an ice axe, ski pole, or wooden stick for balance. Although causing more pain, the decision to walk out may be safer than waiting for help.

Upper Extremities
SHOULDER/CLAVICLE

The collarbone (clavicle) is easily seen and felt along its entire length. It may be injured by a direct blow or a fall onto the shoulder.

What to Look For

➤ Local tenderness, swelling, or deformity indicates a fracture.

➤ Tenderness and a bump at the junction of the collarbone and shoulder are usually due to a sprain.

➤ Clavicle fractures are extremely painful, but sprains are not too painful except when trying to lift the arm. In either case, the victim can use the hand in front of the body.

➤ Fractures of the arm bone (humerus) at the shoulder cause severe pain and marked swelling but are often stable.

➤ *Generally, the arm with a fracture is held against the chest wall, whereas with a dislocation, the arm is held away from the body wall.*

➤ The shoulder blade (scapula) can be fractured by a direct blow, causing local pain, tenderness, and muscle spasm.

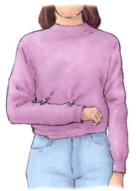
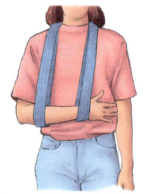

Improvised sling with safety pins   Improvised sling with webbing

What to Do

1. Treat all these injuries with a sling.

2. A sling can be fashioned from any available cloth, or improvised by using safety pins to pin up the arm of a long-sleeved shirt. If the victim is wearing a T-shirt, fold the waist band up over the arm and

pin it to the shirt. A piece of webbing or rope looped around the arm can also make an improvised sling.

3. For better immobilization of fractures or dislocations wrap a swathe around the upper arm and the chest wall after applying a sling.

4. Allow some freedom of the forearm and hand and access to the hand to check circulation, sensation, and movement.

5. A splint can be added to the upper arm for unstable (floppy) fractures of the humerus.

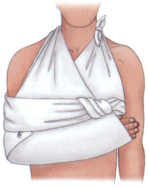

Sling with swathe supporting upper arm against body.

SHOULDER DISLOCATION

Nearly all dislocations of the shoulder joint occur with the arm in the cocked, throwing, or kayak high-brace position with the hand above and behind the shoulder. The head of the humerus is forced out of the socket and lodges in front of the shoulder. A person whose shoulder has dislocated before will recognize when it happens again.

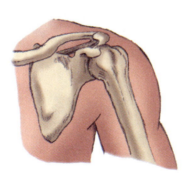
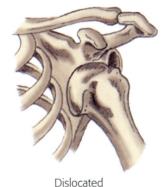

Normal position   Dislocated

What to Look For

➤ The upper arm is usually held away from the body and it is more painful to lay the forearm against the abdomen.

➤ Compare the normal and injured shoulders. With a dislocation, a firm lump is felt in the front of the shoulder hollow, and the side of the shoulder is indented rather than rounded.

➤ Check circulation and sensation of the hand, and also sensation along the outer aspect of the shoulder.

➤ Ask the victim to cock back (extend) the wrist and straighten the fingers and thumb to check the motor nerve function.

➤ Document findings.

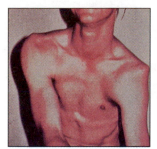

Typical appearance of anterior shoulder dislocation

What to Do

Pull the arm, bent to a right angle at the elbow, steadily out to the side with a strap, jacket, or other material looped around the victim's arm. An assistant pulls in the opposite direction, using straps, a sleeping bag, or clothing around the chest, just below the armpit. You can use muscle relaxation through massage or guided imagery to enhance attempts at relocation.

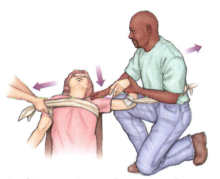

Applying traction on the arm to reduce dislocated shoulder

1. Pad the armpit, chest wall, and front of the elbow, where pressure may be applied during traction.

2. Lean back, using body weight for traction.

3. Gradually elevate the arm to the level of the shoulder while applying traction.

4. Be patient and allow several minutes. Talk to the victim to encourage relaxation.

5. Take 5 to 15 minutes to slowly rotate the arm into a baseball-throwing position.

6. Sometimes you will feel a clunk when the shoulder pops back into its socket; if not, relax traction after a few minutes. If the

shoulder moves freely without pain, it has been reduced. If still unsuccessful, try again but rotate the arm outward, then inward while applying traction, or use a different method, such as the following.

Put the victim face down on a table or flat rock.

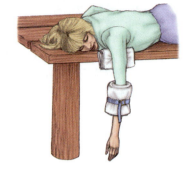

Simple hanging traction to reduce anterior shoulder dislocation

1. Let the arm hang down toward the ground.

2. Position the person and the arm slowly.

3. Tie a 10–15-lb weight to the hand and wrist, using rocks in a day pack or water or sand in a bucket. Do not ask the victim to hold the weight, which would prevent the arm from relaxing. This method is slow (up to an hour) and relaxation is critical, but the muscle will eventually fatigue and allow reduction.

4. After reduction, stabilize the shoulder with sling and swathe.

5. Check circulation and nerve function.

6. The victim can use the hand and forearm, but keep the elbow next to the body and the hand in front to avoid repeat dislocation.

7. For paddlers or climbers who need some motion of the shoulder to travel out of the wilderness, fashion a tether to limit motion of the upper arm.

8. If reduction attempts are not successful, use a sling and swathe with clothing wadded beneath the arm to support it in a comfortable position.

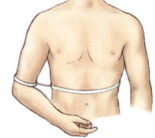

Wrap straps around waist and upper arm to avoid redislocation.

9. Evacuate a victim with an unreduced shoulder.

UPPER ARM
What to Look For

➤ Look for swelling and deformities and feel the shaft of the humerus along its inner aspect.

➤ Most fractures of the bone shaft are unstable and deform or angulate, causing severe pain.

➤ Ask the victim to cock back (extend) the wrist and open and close the fist to check motor nerve function; document for future reference.

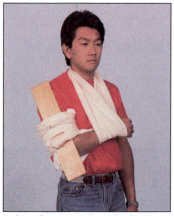 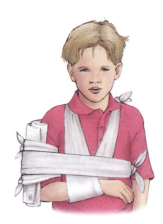

Splinted upper arm with sling, swathe, and padding between the arm and the chest

What to Do

1. Remove any rings because the hand may swell later (see page 129).

2. Splint by stabilizing the arm against the body wall.

3. Place padding between the arm and chest, then wrap the upper arm against the body.

4. You may place a rigid splint on the outside of the arm.

5. Use a sling, but it may be more comfortable to leave the elbow free and dependent.

6. Loop a strap around the wrist and neck to allow the arm to hang in the sling position. Gravity will then provide gentle traction.

ELBOW

The elbow can be injured by a fall directly on the joint or on the outstretched hand.

What to Look For

➤ Major deformities indicate an elbow dislocation or a fracture of the lower humerus.

What to Do

1. Remove any rings because the hand may swell (see page 129).

2. Immobilize with a sling, with the elbow bent as comfort allows.

3. For increased comfort and stability, add a splint along the posterior side from below the shoulder to the wrist.

ADVANCED PROCEDURE   **TRACTION FOR A DISLOCATED ELBOW**

If circulation is obstructed (cool, bluish hand, no pulse at the wrist, numb hand, and unable to move fingers) or help is many hours away, attempt to improve the alignment. Otherwise, splint it in the position in which it is found.

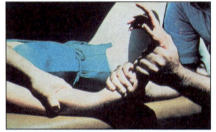

- Apply slow, steady traction to the wrist and forearm with the elbow partially bent (usually how it is found). An assistant applies countertraction to the upper arm.

- If no one else is available to help, put one hand on the upper arm and grasp the wrist with the other hand.

Reduction of elbow dislocation

- A dislocation can usually be reduced without strong pull, but deformed fractures may be only slightly improved at best.

LOWER ARM

What to Look For

➤ The forearm or wrist may be fractured by a fall on the outstretched hand, resulting in a deformity (see page 109).

What to Do

1. Remove rings (see page 129).

2. Attempt to straighten marked angulation of the forearm. While one person holds the arm just above or below the elbow, a second first aider grasps the hand and pulls firmly. If only one rescuer is available, grasp above the elbow and push up while pulling down.

3. Apply a splint to immobilize the hand, wrist, and forearm.

4. Leave the fingers free or wrapped in the functional position (as if holding a ball, glass, or can) with a rolled-up sock, glove, or other soft material in the palm.

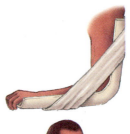

5. For maximal immobilization and comfort, include the elbow in a splint bent to a right angle (90° of flexion).

6. Exercise the fingers to help circulation and reduce swelling.

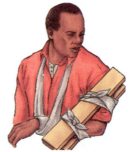

7. For pain and swelling of the lower arm without deformity, apply a splint from the middle of the palm to just below the elbow. A splint on the palm side of the hand and forearm allows the elbow to bend and the arm to rotate, which may be painful. A splint that wraps around the

Splinting for injuries of the elbow or near the elbow when a sling does not provide adequate support

back of the elbow and extends to the back of the hand allows some bending at the elbow, but prevents rotation of the hand and forearm. Simple splints can also be made by folding and rolling a foam ground pad or padding the forearm with clothing or foam pad and sandwiching with any straight firm materials (stays from backpack, pieces of wood, etc.). If the thumb hurts when moved, include it in the splint.

8. Seek medical care if still painful after several days.

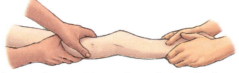

Reduction of forearm fracture. Use similar technique for fractures near wrist.

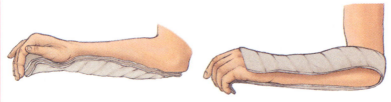

Splinting forearm and wrist using a SAM™ splint

HAND
What to Look For

➤ Deformities and swelling—compare with the uninjured hand.

➤ Carefully note (and draw) the appearance of any deformity to assist future treatment.

What to Do

1. Place the injured hand in the "position of function" (hand will look like it is holding a baseball) by placing a rolled pair of socks in the palm.

2. Attach a rigid splint along the forearm and under the hand.

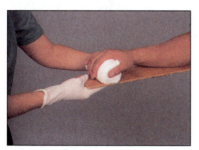 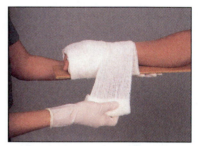

Splinting the hand for fractures in the palm of the hand (metacarpals) or base of the fingers

FINGER
What to Look For

➤ The first joint beyond the knuckle is commonly injured when the finger is bent back or jammed.

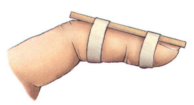

Splint for mallet finger

➤ There is mild swelling, restricted movement, and bruising on the palm side of the joint.

➤ The end joint also can be sprained with rupture of the tendon that straightens the end of the finger (mallet finger). The fingertip is bent and cannot be actively straightened, but is easily pushed up.

➤ Falls on the outstretched hand, as in skiing, bend back the thumb, frequently injuring the ligament on the inner side of the first joint. Pain and inability to grasp or pinch can make simple tasks impossible.

What to Do

Immediately after injury, dislocations of the fingers can be reduced with only minimal discomfort.

1. Grasp the end of the finger in one hand, using gauze or cloth to avoid slipping.

2. Pull steadily and firmly on the partially bent finger, then push the base of the dislocated segment back in place. Remove any rings (see step 7).

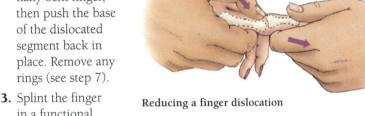

Reducing a finger dislocation

3. Splint the finger in a functional position.

4. For unstable and painful fractures at the base of the finger or the bones in the palm of the hand tape the injured finger to its neighbor, place a soft roll of material in the palm, and then wrap the whole with an elastic bandage, roller gauze, or torn strips of clothing.

5. For fractures of the middle segment of the finger or dislocations on either side, reduce and splint to an adjacent finger ("buddy taping").

6. Place gauze between the fingers to absorb moisture and tape the fingers together in the "position of function."

7. If the person cannot tolerate any movement, add a rigid splint or bulky wrap. After any significant injury to the arm or hand, especially if immobilization is needed, the hand may swell. Remove rings to assure that circulation to the finger is not impaired by swelling. If already swollen or ring cannot be removed, try elevating the arm, applying a cold pack to the finger and soap for lubrication. If still unsuccessful, wrap the finger with dental floss or fishing line as illustrated to remove ring. If still unsuccessful and ring is becoming painfully tight, use the file on a pocket knife to cut the ring.

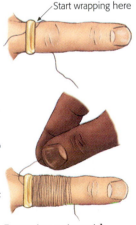

Start wrapping here

Removing a ring with string

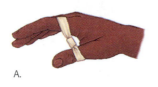

A.

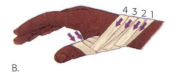

B.

Taping for sprained thumb
A. simplest technique for mild sprain
B. more secure taping for functional support
C. most secure but cannot use thumb

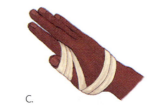

C.

8. Two hand dislocations are difficult to reduce in the field: the base of the index finger and the thumb. Make only one attempt, then immobilize the joint in a functional position.

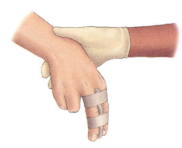

Buddy taping

9. Tape a finger to its neighbor—"buddy tape"—to allow functional support of finger after reducing a finger dislocation or for a sprained finger. For less movement, pad between the fingers and wrap or tape together without space between. Alternatively, splint the middle joint for comfortable function. For a mallet finger, apply a short splint to hold the finger straight.

10. Thumb—For comfort, fashion a splint that includes the thumb and wrist; for best function, try taping. A small chip of bone may be broken off, but urgent evacuation is not necessary.

Lower Extremities
HIP
What to Look For

➤ Diagnosis of a hip fracture is usually easy. Suspect a fracture if a victim has suffered serious injury with pain around the hip that is made more severe with minimal bending or twisting of the hip.

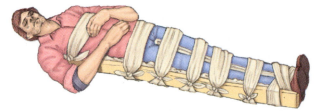

Splint for hip or femur fracture. Note padding under splint and between legs.
Splint extends to armpit to prevent hip movement. Possible splint material:
board, ski, paddle, or oar. Tie legs together with padding between legs.

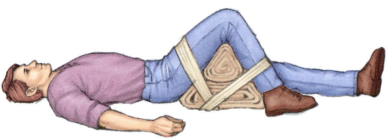

Stabilize a hip injury in the position it is found.

➤ The person is unable to bear weight and lies with the foot rotated
outward.

What to Do

1. Plan to carry the victim out on a litter or sled.

2. Do not put suspected fractures of the hip in traction.

3. Splint the affected leg to the uninjured leg.

4. For greater stabilization, secure a splint using a long board, oar, or
   ski along the side of the body and leg from the armpit to the heel.

5. Put padding between the legs and around the injured leg.

6. For a dislocated hip, evacuate. Dislocations of the hip are unusual.
   There is severe pain, and the hip and knee are held bent with the knee
   turned inward. Since reduction is very difficult, do not attempt it.

PELVIS
What to Look For

➤ Major falls may fracture the pelvis.

➤ Pressing the affected area or squeezing the pelvis side to side or back to front is painful.

➤ Minor fractures around the pubic bone might tolerate walking, but with pain.

➤ Walking, and even sitting, are unbearable after major pelvic fractures.

➤ Pelvic fractures can cause internal bleeding leading to shock.

➤ Check for blood in the urine or inability to urinate due to bladder or urethral injury.

What to Do

1. Stabilize the victim on a rigid backboard, litter, or sled; then evacuate.

UPPER LEG

A victim with a femoral shaft fracture can lose more than a quart of blood into the thigh and, if the fracture is not stabilized, this bleeding can continue.

What to Look For

➤ Fractures of the upper leg (femur) are unstable and have obvious swelling.

What to Do

1. Begin manual traction to the extremity by grasping the ankle and maintaining straight pull on the leg. Traction decreases blood loss, relieves pain, stabilizes fracture fragments, prevents converting a closed fracture into an open fracture, and reduces further soft-tissue damage.

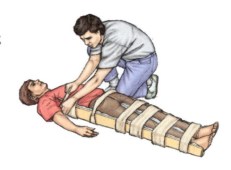

Splinting a femur

2. Manual traction is tiring, but it is possible to construct a splint that provides traction on the leg. Improvising a traction splint can be challenging but is well worth learning for those who plan to increase their skills beyond the introductory level. If needed, design and test a traction splint on an uninjured person.

3. If the victim needs to be moved without traction, stabilize in the position of maximum comfort by splinting the injured to the uninjured leg.
  • Pad between the legs and under the knees to produce a slight bend.
  • For greater support, add a rigid splint from the armpit to below the heel, as for a hip fracture

4. Monitor circulation beyond the injury.
  • Loosen the laces, but do not remove the boot and sock in cold weather. The toe of the boot may be cut away to help monitor circulation.

KNEE

A kneecap (patella) fracture can result from a fall directly on the knee. A severe bruise may cause similar symptoms.

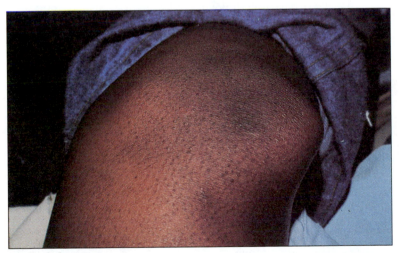

Patella dislocation

What to Look For

➤ Bending or straightening the knee is painful without help lifting the lower leg.

➤ Feel for a gap or marked tenderness along the edges of the kneecap that suggests a fracture.

➤ Dislocation of the kneecap is caused by a pivoting injury with a partially bent knee. The patella is displaced to the outside (laterally) with the knee held bent (in flexion) (see photo page 133).

➤ Major deformity at the knee, other than dislocation of the patella, indicates a serious injury with fracture or dislocation of the leg bones.

➤ The most common injuries to the knee are sprains or tears of the ligaments. Swelling may give the knee a rounded look.

➤ Tenderness is most common on the inner (medial) side of the knee.

➤ The person holds the knee slightly bent.

➤ Pivoting movements cause pain and the knee may feel as if it will "give out."

➤ Weight bearing is usually possible, with the knee held stiffly.

What to Do

1. **Patella dislocation**
   • Flex the hip slightly to relax the thigh muscle, then gently straighten the knee. As the knee is extended, the patella will usually reduce itself. If not, with the knee straight, push the patella back into place with pressure on the outside edge.
   • Wrap the leg in a cylinder splint made from a foam sleeping pad, or sandwich on both sides with a rigid splint. This will stabilize the knee, and the person may be able to walk out unaided.
   • Improvise a cane or crutch if needed.

2. **Sprains**
   • Wrap the knee firmly with an elastic (ACE™) bandage or cylinder splint as shown here.
   • If supported by a walking stick, the patient may walk. However, walking will be difficult in steep or rugged terrain.

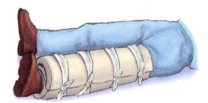

Cylinder splint

3. **Severe pain, major deformity, and moderate to severe swelling**
   • Check for diminished blood flow (cool, bluish foot, no pulses at the ankle, numb foot, and pain on movement of toes).

- If circulation in the foot appears to be poor, attempt to improve alignment with direct traction along the normal long axis of the leg.
- Splint securely but without compromising circulation to the foot.
- If the leg is bent at the knee at a strange angle, realign the leg. This is easier than splinting at odd angles.
- Do not ask the victim to stand or walk.
- Evacuate.

LOWER LEG

The shinbone (tibia) can easily be felt under the skin along the front and inner side of the lower leg.

What to Look For

➤ Fractures are generally obvious with severe pain, early swelling, instability, some deformity, and inability to bear any weight.

➤ Tibial fractures often puncture the skin, creating an open fracture.

➤ Isolated tenderness and pain on the outer aspect of the leg with no tenderness of the shinbone may be a fibula fracture (smaller bone on the outer side of the leg).

What to Do

1. Correct angular deformities with gentle traction at the ankle as illustrated in the section on ankle injuries.

2. Splint lower leg fractures to immobilize the knee and ankle. Use any padded materials to secure the leg and prevent the ankle and knee from movement. Provide support with a small pad under the knee.

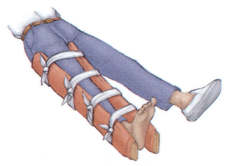

Splint for lower leg (tibia and fibula fracture)

Wrap the leg first in a sleeping pad. Hold the foot and provide traction on the leg while another person applies the splint.

3. Traction splinting is not generally done for lower leg fractures. However, manual traction can be used to further reduce pain, muscle spasm, and bleeding while applying a splint.

4. Evacuate.

5. If the fibula alone is fractured with the tibia intact, the victim can walk with a cane or crutch and ankle support.

ANKLE

Most ankle injuries are sprains of the outside (lateral) ligaments, caused by the foot turning inward. It is difficult to tell the difference between a severe sprain and a fracture. Ligament injuries and fractures often occur together, and dislocations are nearly always associated with multiple fractures. Treat as a fracture whenever there is diffuse, marked swelling, inability to bear weight, or obvious signs of fracture, such as a deformity or crepitus (crunching with movement).

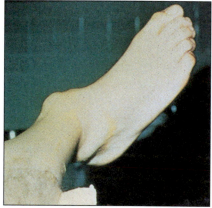

Ankle fracture/dislocation

What to Look For

➤ The typical sprained ankle is swollen, tender, and bruised around the knob of bone on the outer side of the ankle (lateral malleolus).

➤ To determine whether an ankle is sprained or fractured,
  • Press gently along the bones. Pain and marked tenderness over the bones at either the back edge or tip of either ankle bone (malleolus) or the outside bone of the foot (metatarsal) suggest a fracture.
  • Ask the victim if he or she tried standing on the injured ankle. Putting weight on the ankle may hurt, but if the victim is able to take four or more steps, the ankle is probably only sprained or has a minor fracture. Inability to walk does not necessarily mean there is a fracture.

What to Do

1. Decide whether to remove the boot or leave it on: Remove the boot both for examination and treatment or if the foot is wet. **However, if you take off the boot, you may not get it back on;** so leave it on if the person needs to walk or you are in severe weather or difficult terrain.

2. Check the foot's circulation, sensation, and movement (see page 111).

3. Reduce and straighten any deformity of the ankle. Tight, stretched overlying skin is in danger of breaking down. Hold the toes and back of the heel, lift the leg, and apply traction. Improved alignment results without much effort.

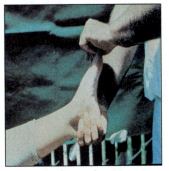

4. Use the RICE procedures (see page 115). The goal of RICE is to limit swelling.

Technique for applying traction to reduce ankle or straighten lower leg fracture

5. For sprained ankle, wrap with an elastic bandage in figure-8 pattern, or simple overlapping, from toes of foot, upward. For extra compression, add a **U**-shaped pad (made of rolled bandana, piece of ground foam, or other material) around the outer knob of the ankle. For a mild sprain, taping the ankle will provide enough support to reduce swelling but will allow walking.

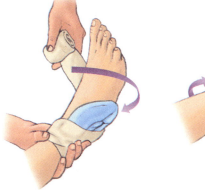
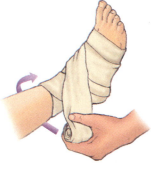

Compression wrap for a sprained ankle

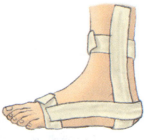

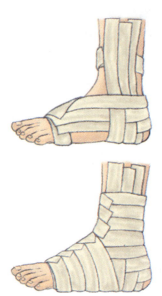

Ankle taping can provide excellent support and allow use of a sprained ankle.

6. Splint ankle fractures with a parka, foam sleeping pad, SAM™ splint, or pillow arranged in a **U**-shape around the foot and lower leg. With less severe ankle injuries, if the ankle is supported by splint or tape, and pain is bearable, the victim may be able to walk.

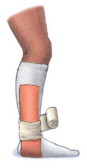

A SAM™ splint.

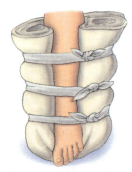

A foam sleeping pad in a U-shape will immobilize the foot and ankle.

FOOT

Fractures of the long bones of the foot (metatarsals) may occur from dropping a heavy object on the foot or from the stress of sustained hiking.

What to Look For

➤ local tenderness and pain with walking

➤ swelling, bruising, and pain caused by a blow to the foot

What to Do

1. A stiff-sole boot and cane or crutch will allow the person to walk.

2. If pain increases with walking, the person should not continue. Evacuate.

TOES

Toes may be fractured by stubbing them while walking without shoes.

What to Look For

➤ Compare injured and uninjured sides.

What to Do

1. If a toe has a different bend or angle compared to the same toe on the other foot, pull straight outward to put back into normal position.

2. Immobilize an injured toe by buddy-taping it to its neighbor with padding in between.

3. Walking is allowed. A stiff-sole boot may be more comfortable than a soft shoe.

Spine

The spine is a column of vertebrae extending from the base of the skull to the tailbone. Each vertebra is a bony ring through which the spinal cord passes. The spinal cord is made up of long tracts of nerves that join the brain with the rest of the body. If a broken vertebra pinches the spinal cord, paralysis can result. These injuries most often occur from severe accidents when the victim strikes the head or lands on the upper back or buttocks, compressing the spine, or with direct falls onto the spine. This may occur in falls, vehicular crashes with unrestrained victims, or a skier striking a tree head-on. Urban first aid advises not to move victims with potential spinal injury; in the wilderness, however, it may be necessary to move these people for a more thorough evaluation or to move them to a safer place. You also need to decide when to allow a conscious person to get up and move around (see "When to Remove Spinal Immobilization" in this chapter). Full spinal immobilization involves a potentially hazardous, long, and costly rescue.

What to Look For

➤ numbness, tingling, weakness, or burning sensation in arms or legs

➤ loss of bowel or bladder control (inability to urinate)

➤ paralysis of arms and/or legs

➤ tenderness along the midline prominence of the spine

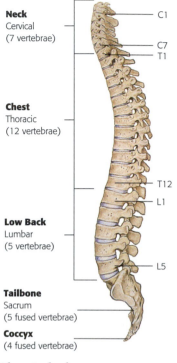

Neck
Cervical
(7 vertebrae)

Chest
Thoracic
(12 vertebrae)

Low Back
Lumbar
(5 vertebrae)

Tailbone
Sacrum
(5 fused vertebrae)

Coccyx
(4 fused vertebrae)

C1

C7
T1

T12

L1

L5

The spinal column

Ask a responsive victim these questions:

➤ Is there pain? Often a victim will describe nerve pain as an "electric shock." The pain from nerve injuries in the neck radiates to the arms; from upper-back injuries, around the ribs; from lower-back injuries, down the legs. Similar symptoms that develop without a fall might be due to a herniated disk.

➤ Can you move your feet? Ask the victim to move the foot, pushing downward and upward against your hand despite pain in the back or other areas. If a good effort produces no movement or very weak movement, the victim may have injured the spinal cord.

➤ Can you move your fingers? Ask the victim to grip your hand. A strong grip, equal on both sides, indicates that a spinal cord injury is unlikely; but weak or absent grip on one or both sides indicates a possible spinal cord injury in the neck.

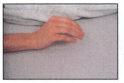

1. Victim wiggles fingers

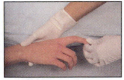

2. Rescuer touches fingers or tests ability to feel light prick with safety pin

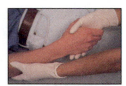

3. Victim squeezes rescuer's hand

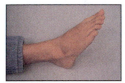

4. Victim wiggles toes

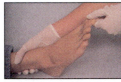

5. Rescuer touches toes

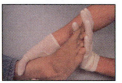

6. Victim pushes foot against rescuer's hand

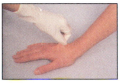

7. Pinch hand

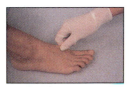

8. Pinch foot

Checking for spinal injuries

For an unresponsive victim:

➤ Ask bystanders what happened. If there was a significant fall, blow to the head, or diving injury, assume that the victim has a spinal injury until a good evaluation shows otherwise.

➤ Look for injuries around the head and spine (cuts, bruises, and deformities).

➤ Pinch the victim's hands (either palm or back) and foot (sole or top of the bare foot). A lack of reaction to painful stimuli could mean spinal cord damage.

What to Do

1. Check the ABCs (see chapter 3).

2. Tell the person to remain still. If the victim has spinal pain, is unresponsive, or is confused following a head injury, stabilize the spine, especially the neck, to avoid further damage. The ribs

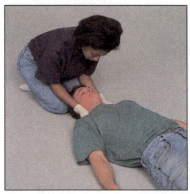 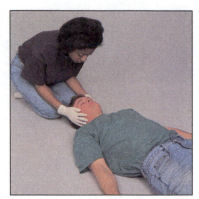

Manual immobilization of cervical spine options

stabilize the thoracic spine and the large muscles of the lumbar area stabilize the lower spine.

3. Tell a responsive and cooperative victim not to move. To stabilize the neck initially, grasp the victim's collarbone (clavicle) and shoulder (trapezius muscle) and cradle the head between the insides of your forearms. If the victim is sitting upright, support the head with your hands. Hold the head and neck still and lower the victim slowly to the back. There should be no need to manipulate the neck into an uncomfortable position: a conscious, sober person will try to protect a painful neck from damaging movements.

4. Hold the head still (support using rocks padded with clothing or similar objects) while improvising better immobilization.

5. A short spine board can be improvised from a backpack, life jacket, paddles, ski board, snowshoe, or snow shovel.

6. Place the "board" behind the head, neck, and chest with rolled clothing on either side of the head to prevent rotation, and padding beneath the back of the head.

7. The head and neck should be in the neutral position, with the eyes looking straight forward and the nose in line with the navel.

8. Secure the trunk firmly to the board around the chest, below the arms, and around the forehead. A similar partial spine board can be used for the lumbar or thoracic spine.

9. A simple neck collar can be fashioned from an aluminum foam splint (SAM™ splint), a rolled jacket or towel, or a padded hip belt from a backpack. A neck collar alone is not adequate for immobilizing someone with a high suspicion of serious neck injury, but can be used for comfort after a strain or after waking up with a painful neck.

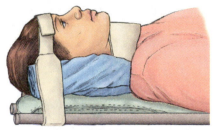

Improvised immobilization of cervical spine

Moving a Victim with a Spinal Injury

A victim in an awkward position after a fall, wedged between trees or rocks, or lying face-down should be extricated and placed on the back with the spine straight (see chapter 2). Straighten the head and neck of an unconscious victim to maintain an open airway. Injured persons may need to be moved to a secure place where you can provide further first aid. If you are alone, correctly moving a victim with suspected spinal injury without a litter or backboard is impossible. Be especially cautious if there are any of the neurologic signs mentioned above. To place a backboard under a victim assign one person to control the head and neck and to give the commands for any movement to other rescuers. This person cradles the head between the insides of the forearms while holding onto the top of the shoulder, or simply holds the head and jaw firmly with a hand on either side. Gently straighten the head

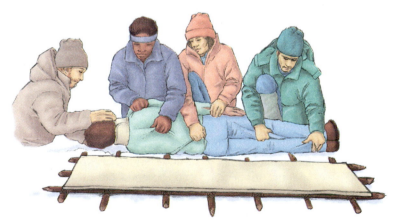

Log-roll technique

and neck if necessary. To examine the back and spine, to turn onto the back, or to place on an improvised backboard, roll the victim like a log, with no twisting or bending. Lifting requires one or more rescuers on each side to support the chest, pelvis, and legs, and one at the head.

When to Remove Spinal Immobilization

In the wilderness, seek a balance between the difficulties and dangers of evacuating an immobilized victim and the risks of not immobilizing a spine injury. Fortunately, spine injuries are rare.

To exclude a spine injury in a victim with a potential injury (fall, blow to the head, or diving injury) use the following criterion:

If the victim fails a step in the evaluation, immobilize until help and better equipment can be obtained.

Spinal immobilization is *not* needed if

- the victim has calmed down from the initial reaction to injury and is fully alert, cooperative, and *not* intoxicated

- there are no signs or symptoms of spinal cord injury (numbness, tingling, burning sensation in arms or legs; paralysis or weakness of fingers, toes, hands, feet, unless explained by injury to that part)

- there is no marked tenderness when pressing on the spine (not including muscles on either side of the spine)

- there is no marked muscle spasm (may develop hours later or next day if there has been a sprain/strain)

- there is no severe midline spine pain with movement (exclude muscle tightness to side of spine and extending along top and inside of shoulder blade)

- there are no other painful injuries that could make the spine difficult to evaluate (e.g., multiple broken ribs, fractures of the arms or legs, or major injury close to the spine)

In the event that signs and symptoms listed above do not suggest spine injury, you can support the head and have the victim rotate then bend the neck slowly through normal range of motion. You can then support the victim in an attempt to sit and stand, then slowly try rotation, side, and forward bending. Mild soreness only, with minimal limitation of motion, indicates no serious spine injury.

Guidelines for Evacuation of Musculoskeletal Injuries

Evacuate, as rapidly as possible, for

- open fractures
- injuries with nerve damage or compromised blood supply not alleviated by realignment
- injuries with suspected spinal cord damage
- injuries associated with serious blood loss
- major fractures (hip, femur, pelvis, injury with deformity at the knee, ankle, elbow)
- major dislocations or those that cannot be relocated

Provide nonurgent or assisted evacuation for injuries that cause sufficient pain or disability so that the person cannot safely or effectively continue travel.

Evacuation is unnecessary for

- digit (finger or toe) injuries
- minimal injuries to other joints
- suspected fractures with no deformity or dislocations after reduction when splinting provides comfort and adequate function, and function is adequate to continue safely

Circulatory Emergencies

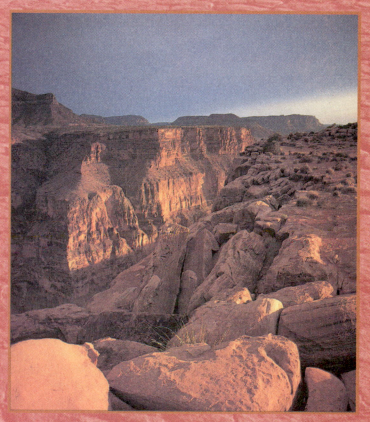

Anatomy and Physiology • Shock •

Heart Disease and Chest Pain

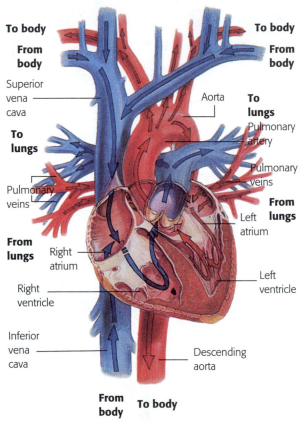

To body

From body

Superior vena cava

To lungs

Pulmonary veins

From lungs

Right atrium

Right ventricle

Inferior vena cava

Aorta

To lungs

Pulmonary artery

Pulmonary veins

From lungs

Left atrium

Left ventricle

To body

From body

Descending aorta

From body **To body**

Diagram of the heart

Anatomy and Physiology

There are three components to the circulatory system: the heart, blood vessels, and blood.

The heart is a four-chambered muscular pump that receives oxygen-deficient blood from the body; pumps it through the lungs, where the blood gets rid of carbon dioxide and refills with oxygen; then pumps oxygen-rich blood to the body. Heart function is variable, with the capacity to slow down during periods of rest and accelerate during exercise or stress to meet the demands of the body.

Blood vessels are reactive tubes for carrying red cells and plasma, the fluid component of blood. Arteries carry blood away from the heart to the tissues, and veins carry blood back to the heart. As arteries get farther away from the heart they decrease in size and eventually become a network of microscopically small capillaries. It is through the capillaries that the exchange of oxygen and carbon dioxide takes place, with oxygen passing into the tissues and carbon dioxide passing back into the blood. The blood then travels through veins, which become larger as they approach the heart. The smaller blood vessels have the ability to dilate or contract in response to numerous stimuli, particularly heat and cold.

Blood is a suspension of cells in a protein-rich fluid. Red cells, which carry oxygen, make up most of the cells; white cells defend the body against infections; and platelets are essential for clotting.

The circulatory system works at its best only when all the parts are functioning well: a healthy heart, normal blood volume, enough red cells to carry oxygen, and blood vessels that are neither overly dilated nor excessively contracted.

The most likely emergencies encountered in the wilderness are: shock, resulting from blood loss, anaphylaxis, and severe dehydration; and heart disease, including angina, heart attack, and abnormal heart rhythms.

Shock

Shock occurs when blood flow is inadequate to maintain the supply of oxygen. Oxygen, the fuel of life, is carried by the red blood cells from the lungs to all living tissues in the body. The two most important causes of shock are low blood volume and low blood pressure. Loss of 1 to 1½ pints in an adult may cause the first stages of shock.

1. Low blood volume can result from
   - internal or external blood loss (internal blood loss usually occurs in the abdomen—see chapter 12)
   - severe dehydration due to diarrhea, vomiting, or sweating, especially if combined with a lack of fluid intake
   - dilation of the blood vessels, as in anaphylaxis (see chapter 13) or with spinal cord damage: small blood vessels dilate and the blood volume is insufficient to fill the enlarged space, causing blood pressure to fall

2. Low blood pressure may be due to the inability of the heart to pump blood, as after a heart attack. Damaged heart muscle cannot pump effectively; blood flow and blood pressure fall to dangerous levels.

3. Severe infections can produce toxins that cause shock.

DO NOT

- confuse true shock with emotional "shock." True shock may be fatal; emotional shock is not usually dangerous. Fainting results from a brief drop in blood pressure and is preceded by some of the signs of shock, but is usually harmless and temporary (see chapter 11).

What to Look For

➤ rapid, weak pulse; this is the most consistent sign of shock. When blood volume is reduced, the heart speeds up, trying to compensate by circulating the blood more rapidly; blood pressure falls. The faint pulse is due to low blood pressure. In early shock the pulse rate may be normal when the victim is lying down, but speeds up when the person sits or stands.

➤ rapid breathing; breathing also speeds up to supply more oxygen to the blood

➤ weak pulse, the result of low blood pressure

➤ pale or bluish (cyanotic) skin, nail beds, and lips. Blood vessels in the skin constrict, redirecting blood flow to more vital organs and producing changes in skin color and temperature.

➤ damp, clammy skin

➤ restlessness, anxiety, weakness

➤ nausea and vomiting

➤ altered level of responsiveness

Shock requires hospital treatment. Do not expect true shock to improve spontaneously. Your treatment will reduce the effects, at best.

What to Do

1. Check the ABCs and examine the individual, both front and back, for bleeding. If external bleeding seems insufficient to cause shock, consider internal bleeding into the abdomen, chest, stomach, or intestines.

2. Control all bleeding and treat any major injuries.

3. Lay the victim on his or her back with the feet elevated 8 to 12 inches, to increase blood flow from the legs to the heart.

4. Keep the victim sheltered and warm. Use spare clothes, coats, blankets, or sleeping bags over and under the victim to prevent heat loss.

5. Do not give food to a victim in traumatic shock. If the person is able to swallow, give only clear liquids.

6. If shock is due to dehydration, give water and electrolyte replacement solutions orally. Large volumes may be required (see appendix D).

7. Treat a severely injured person as if shock is inevitable.

8. Evacuate as quickly as possible.

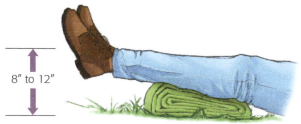

8" to 12"

Raise legs of victim in shock.

PEDIATRIC NOTE Children respond to shock by increasing the heart rate. The normal maximum heart rate for infants is 160/min.; for preschool children 140/min.; and for school age children 120/min. The pulse can also be elevated due to pain or fear. The blood pressure in a child who is bleeding will be maintained until approximately 40% of the blood volume has been lost. The unwary first aider may get false comfort from an apparently normal, strong pulse. After 40% of the blood volume has been lost, a child's condition deteriorates rapidly. An increasing pulse rate, prolonged capillary refill time, and diminishing consciousness are signs of impending shock. A restless, lethargic child, especially in the presence of parents, may be underoxygenated due to undetected blood loss. Monitor the vital signs and alertness to detect impending shock before the situation turns critical.

INTERNAL BLEEDING

Internal bleeding comes from disorders such as stomach ulcers, miscarriages, and injuries that do not break the skin (e.g., injuries to the lung that bleed into the chest, or injuries to the spleen or liver that bleed into the abdominal cavity). Fractures of the pelvis, hip, or thigh also can result in serious hidden bleeding. Since no blood is seen, internal bleeding can be difficult to detect, can seldom be controlled in the field, and may be life-threatening.

What to Look For

➤ a painful, tender, rigid abdomen (possible bleeding into the abdomen)

➤ fractured ribs or bruises on the chest; shortness of breath

➤ unexplained signs of shock (weakness, dizziness, or fainting; a rapid pulse; cold, moist skin)

➤ vomiting or coughing up blood

➤ stools that are black or contain large amounts of blood (black color results from digested blood)

➤ vaginal bleeding and/or pain in a pregnant woman (see chapter 14)

What to Do

1. Check the ABCs repeatedly to evaluate the severity of bleeding.

2. Be prepared for vomiting. If the person is not alert, lay the victim on his or her side to prevent inhalation of vomit.

3. If the victim is alert, raise the legs 8 to 12 inches to treat shock and keep the person warm.

4. Evacuate to medical care immediately.

Heart Disease and Chest Pain

Consider serious disease when chest pain is associated with shortness of breath, weakness, cyanosis, and cold, clammy skin; is heavy, crushing, burning, or squeezing pain beneath the breastbone; radiates to the neck, jaw, throat, arms, or shoulders; or occurs in a person with a history of heart or lung disease with previous attacks of similar pain.

The pain of heart disease is heavy, dull, burning, squeezing, or crushing, rather than sharp. It is substernal—located under the breastbone— rather than in the left chest "over the heart." It frequently radiates to the throat, neck, jaw, left shoulder, or left arm, and occasionally to the right shoulder, right arm, or upper back. Someone who complains of indigestion brought on by exercise may really have heart disease.

The cause of most heart pain is coronary artery disease. Cholesterol deposits narrow the coronary arteries and block the supply of blood to the heart muscle (myocardium). If the narrowing is minor, the person may be able to perform everyday activities without difficulty. During exercise or strong emotion, however, more blood is needed by the heart muscle than can pass through the narrowed arteries, and the relative lack of blood to the heart muscle causes pain.

A characteristic story is that the victim walks uphill after a heavy meal and develops crushing central chest pain that brings the person to a halt. After a minute or two of rest, the pain goes away but returns after the victim continues to walk. Pain relieved by rest or nitroglycerine (see below) or lasting less than 15 minutes is called *angina*. More severe, longer-lasting pain not relieved by rest or nitroglycerine may signal that the victim is having a *heart attack*, which is an emergency. The victim is typically anxious, short of breath, has cold, clammy, and/or cyanotic skin, may feel lightheaded, and may prefer to sit rather than lie down. Occasionally, however, the victim may experience little discomfort and may deny that a heart attack is occurring.

What to Look For

Do an initial survey (see chapter 3). Signs that the person is obviously in distress are:

➤ victim's SAMPLE history (see pages 45–46), particularly previous similar pain; a history of heart or lung disease; recent chest injury; unusual physical activity involving the chest muscles (lifting, climbing, paddling, carrying a heavy pack), or a recent respiratory infection. Ask about previous digestive system disease such as ulcer or gallbladder disease, "nervous stomach," hiatus hernia, and irritable bowel disease. Ask about medicines being taken and what they are for.

➤ abnormal pulse; abnormal respirations; altered responsiveness

➤ location, type, severity, and duration of pain; change in pain; possible relation to breathing, coughing, or physical activity; shortness of breath. Ask the victim to *describe the pain*.

➤ symptoms of infection (chills, fever, cough, shortness of breath, sore throat, earache, stuffy head that might suggest a chest infection)

➤ "indigestion"

➤ changes in the vital signs, especially temperature, pulse, breathing rate, and skin characteristics (color, temperature, and moisture)

Note: After an anginal attack the victim may look and feel normal. During a heart attack the victim is nervous, is obviously in pain, and looks sick.

What to Do

For angina pectoris:

1. Suspect angina if typical pain occurs in a middle-aged or elderly person, especially one with a history of known heart disease or angina.

2. If the victim has had previous attacks, the person will usually be carrying nitroglycerine (small, white pills about ½ the size of an aspirin, or a spray), and will know how to use it. Assist the victim in using the medicine according to the directions on the container. Nitroglycerine enlarges the blood vessels and increases blood flow to the heart muscle. *Be sure the victim is sitting or lying down* when taking nitroglycerine because it occasionally causes a drop in blood pressure and often causes a pounding headache.

3. If pain continues, repeat the dose twice at 3-minute intervals.

4. If the pain stops within 15 minutes, it is probably angina. If it continues, suspect a heart attack (see below).

5. Evacuate anyone you suspect has angina. He or she may walk out if able to do so without pain.

If you suspect a heart attack:

1. Shelter the victim and keep him or her warm.

2. Give one aspirin. (Aspirin, given early during a heart attack, reduces mortality.)

3. Give nothing but water or clear, bland liquids to drink.

4. Arrange immediate evacuation.

CHANGES IN CARDIAC RHYTHM

The normal heartbeat is regular in rhythm—sometimes slow and sometimes fast, but always regular. As you feel a pulse you may occasionally feel a "skipped beat"—a break in the regularity of the beat—or total irregularity. Most rhythm irregularities are harmless. Total irregularity (atrial fibrillation, not to be confused with fatal ventricular fibrillation) is sometimes found at high altitude and in victims of hypothermia. In both instances the condition reverts to normal when the person is removed from the contributing environment.

Evacuate the victim if the heart rate is greater than 120 beats per minute at rest and the person is unable to function normally.

CHAPTER 10

Respiratory Emergencies

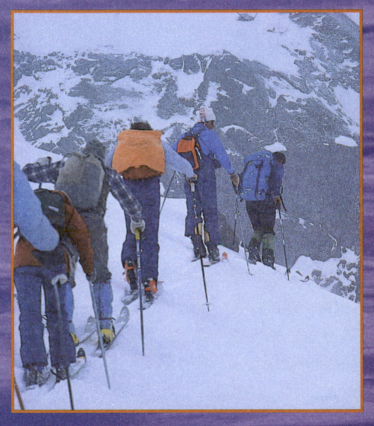

**Anatomy and Physiology • Chest Injury •
Respiratory Illnesses**

The respiratory system brings air into the lungs, where it comes into contact with the blood. In the smallest air sacs (alveoli), oxygen moves across a thin membrane into the red cells of the blood while carbon dioxide moves out of the blood.

The respiratory system includes the nose, pharynx, trachea, bronchi, and alveoli, which serve as air passages. The ribs, chest muscles, and diaphragm provide the pumping mechanism for moving air into and out of the lungs.

Anatomy and Physiology

The chest is bounded by the collarbones above and the lower margin of the ribcage below. There are 12 ribs on each side, attached to the vertebral column posteriorly. The top 10 ribs join the sternum in front, but the eleventh and twelfth ribs are short and do not extend around to the front.

Air enters the chest through the mouth and nose, passes between the vocal cords, and travels down the trachea (windpipe), which divides behind the middle of the breastbone into left and right bronchi, one to each lung.

The main structures within the chest are the two lungs on each side and, in the midline, the heart and large arteries and veins attached to the heart. The lungs are each surrounded by a membrane, the pleura, which also lines the inside of the chest wall. The potential space between each lung and the chest wall, the pleural space, can fill with blood or air after injuries to the lungs or chest wall. It is possible to have blood or air in one pleural space with none in the other. The lungs are kept expanded by a negative pressure in each pleural space. If the pleural space is opened, the partial vacuum is broken and the lungs collapse.

PEDIATRIC NOTE The normal respiratory rate is higher in children than in adults and is age dependent: 30/min. for preschool children; 20/min. for school age children; and 12/min. for adolescents. Difficult labored breathing, and grunting together with a rapid respiratory rate all indicate a problem. The ribs are very resilient in children. A severe direct blow to the chest may fail to fracture ribs, but can produce serious bruising of the lungs and other structures.

The most likely respiratory emergencies in the wilderness are closed and open injuries, and illnesses. Closed injuries include fractured ribs, flail chest, possible contusion of lungs or heart, traumatic pneumothorax (air in the chest), hemothorax (blood in the chest). Open injuries include sucking chest wound, traumatic pneumothorax, penetrating wounds. Illnesses include upper respiratory infections, pneumonia, asthma, nonspecific shortness of breath, and high altitude pulmonary edema (HAPE).

Chest Injury

In a serious accident the head and chest can suffer, but the chest injury may pass unnoticed because of the more obvious head injury. Examine both areas carefully, because injuries to either may be fatal.

The chest may be crushed (closed injury) or punctured (open injury), damaging the chest wall (ribs and muscles), the lung, or both. Preliminary assessment and treatment for either an open or closed chest injury are the same. Be sure to examine the bare chest in adequate light.

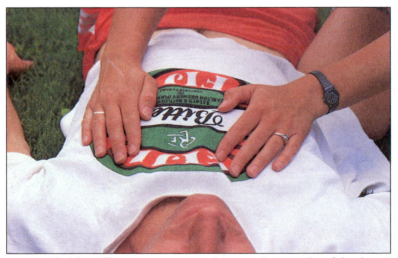

Look and feel for differences in movement between the two sides of the chest.

What to Look For

➤ abnormal breathing or signs of shock; check ABCs

➤ bluish lips, indicating inadequately oxygenated blood

➤ blood-flecked spit, suggesting lung injury

➤ external wounds

➤ decreased movement of the injured side of the chest. Both sides should move equally with each breath. Place your palms flat on the chest, one on each side of the midline; the chest will move less on the injured side.

➤ shallow, irregular, rapid breathing (more than 30 breaths per minute). Painful breathing and coughing may be due to broken ribs or lung damage.

➤ croaking, obstructed breathing; the sound of air moving into or out of a sucking wound

What to Do

1. Keep the airway open.

2. Lay the victim on the injured side; the weight of the body acts as a splint. Put a pad of clothes underneath the body for extra support and for ground insulation.

3. Encourage deep breathing. If breathing is painful, hold the chest wall to help coughing. Inhaling steam may help loosen secretions and make coughing easier.

SINGLE RIB FRACTURES
What to Look For

➤ severe pain, especially on breathing and movement, making breathing shallow and discouraging coughing

➤ grating or clicking at the site of pain and tenderness caused by movement of broken rib ends—a definite sign of fracture

➤ blood in the spit, usually indicating injury to lung unless the blood comes from the nose or throat

What to Do

1. Give painkillers.

2. Do not splint the chest with a tight wrap unless the pain with movement is very bad.

3. A single, simple rib fracture is not an urgent problem and does not require the victim to be evacuated, although carrying a pack will be painful.

MULTIPLE RIB FRACTURES

When several ribs are fractured and the chest wall is pushed in, jagged rib ends may puncture underlying lung, releasing air (pneumothorax) or blood (hemothorax) into the chest cavity. To tell the difference between these two or to treat them in the wilderness is almost impossible.

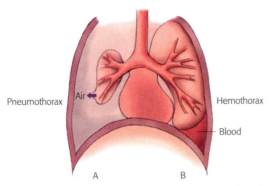

A hemopneumothorax occurs if both blood and air enter pleural space with partial collapse of lung. A. Air escapes from lung, causing collapse of lung. B. Blood from torn lung enters pleural space without collapse of lung.

CLOSED INJURY

Fractures of the lower ribs on the left side may damage the spleen; on the right side, the liver.

If several ribs are broken in two places, *paradoxical breathing* can occur—a segment of the chest wall will move in the opposite direction to the rest of the chest during breathing (sucking in on inspiration, when the chest normally expands, and bulging on expiration, when the chest deflates). This is known as a *flail chest.* The lungs are poorly ventilated, the exchange of gases in the lungs diminishes, and the victim becomes cyanotic (blue).

What to Look For

➤ shortness of breath. Increasing shortness of breath may signify an associated lung injury, pneumothorax or hemothorax, or flail chest.

➤ tenderness over the broken ribs

➤ tenderness just below the lower ribs, indicating a possible abdominal injury

> pain in the shoulder, possibly due to blood under the diaphragm

> signs of shock from internal bleeding

> air under the skin—a spongy, crackling feeling over the affected side (subcutaneous emphysema), indicating an air leak into the chest wall from a torn lung

What to Do

1. Evacuate urgently. Someone with multiple rib fractures will not be able to continue a trip.

2. If a segment of chest appears to move abnormally, support it with a heavy dressing or a large bag filled with earth, bandaged firmly in position.

3. Have the victim lie on the affected side; this may reduce pain and help breathing by splinting the injury.

OPEN INJURY

This is an open wound large enough to permit air to flow in and out of the chest with each breath. The lung collapses and cannot be expanded until the wound is sealed.

What to Look For

> injury after a severe blow or fall

> broken skin, with an obvious hole in the chest wall through which air moves noisily during both inhalation and exhalation

What to Do

1. Seal an open, sucking wound with a thick, impermeable dressing (petroleum jelly on gauze and a bulky dressing, or improvised with a plastic bag or kitchen wrap padded with bulky cloth) taped closely to the skin to prevent escape or entry of air. Sometimes sealing the wound is harmful. If there is a tear in the lung in addition to the wound in the chest wall, air may continue to escape into the pleural space and build up pressure.

2. If the victim's condition becomes worse, release a corner of the dressing to allow escape of air with expiration.

PNEUMOTHORAX OR HEMOTHORAX

Air enters the chest cavity (pleural space) from outside through a penetrating wound or from the surface of the lung torn by a fractured rib.

Air can also enter the pleural space spontaneously in a healthy young person by rupture of a small bleb (blister) on the surface of the lung. The vacuum normally present in the chest cavity is broken and the lung collapses.

The first-aider cannot do anything other than recognize that the victim has a severe respiratory problem, and arrange immediate evacuation. If the pneumothorax is severe and the lung totally collapsed, it may be obvious that the affected side is not moving as well as the normal side.

What to Look For

➤ no injury visible; one side of the chest moving less than the other because of voluntary "splinting"

What to Do

1. Allow the person to adopt the most comfortable position that does not hinder breathing.

2. Evacuate immediately.

TENSION PNEUMOTHORAX

A flaplike tear on the surface of the lung may act as a one-way valve. Air is sucked into the pleural space with each breath, but the flap-valve closes on expiration. More and more air is trapped in the pleural space. The pressure within the chest increases rapidly, with serious and immediate effects on the functions of the lung and heart. If the person appears to be dying, act urgently—*tension pneumothorax kills quickly.*

What to Look For

➤ gasping, labored breathing, with heaving chest and neck muscles

➤ increased blueness of lips and fingernails

➤ less movement of the affected side of the chest than of the normal side

TENSION PNEUMOTHORAX   ADVANCED PROCEDURE

What to Do

The following medical procedure is the only hope of saving life and is beyond the scope of standard first aid.

1. Push a large medical needle or catheter into the affected chest cavity to allow air to escape and to relieve pressure within the chest.
2. Evacuate immediately.

Respiratory Illnesses
CHEST PAIN

Chest pain is common and usually not due to serious disease, but should never be ignored because it may occasionally signal life-threatening illness. The cause may be obscure and difficult to discover even in a hospital. Chest pain causes anxiety because of its association with heart trouble. Most chest pain is caused by one of the following:

* irritation of ribs, muscles, or joints in the chest wall
* heart disease
* respiratory disease
* gastrointestinal disease

CHEST WALL PAIN

Exercise or a minor injury can sprain or bruise ribs, chest muscles, or the joints between the ribs and the breastbone. The person can point to the site of the pain, which is tender on examination. The pain is aching or sharp and aggravated by deep breathing, coughing, twisting the trunk, or moving the arms and shoulders.

RESPIRATORY PAIN DUE TO DISEASE

Respiratory pain can be a raw feeling in the throat, neck, or beneath the breastbone; an ache in the front of the chest; or a stabbing pain in one side of the chest aggravated by coughing or deep breathing. A likely candidate is a person who already has a head or chest cold. Pain in the throat may be aggravated by swallowing; pain in the neck or beneath the breastbone may be aggravated by coughing.

PNEUMONIA AND PLEURISY

Victims with pneumonia or pleurisy are sick—with fever, shaking chills, and a severe cough that produces yellow or green sputum. They are frequently short of breath and occasionally have blood in the sputum. Chest pain tends to be one-sided and aggravated by coughing or breathing. Occasionally, pain in the lower chest is due to disease of organs that lie close under the diaphragm.

SHORTNESS OF BREATH

Someone with shortness of breath works hard to obtain enough air. Breaths may be too slow, too fast, or too shallow, and frequently too fast and too shallow at the same time.

Shortness of breath during hard physical work or on first arriving at high altitude is natural and harmless, even for a fit person, unless it is out of proportion to the effort.

The causes of shortness of breath are usually in the respiratory system or heart. Some persons say they are short of breath when they mean they have a stuffy nose.

What to Look For

➤ the three most common respiratory symptoms—pain, cough, shortness of breath

➤ location, type, severity, and duration of pain; changes in pain; its relation to breathing, coughing, physical activity, eating, twisting the trunk, or moving the arms

➤ the victim's SAMPLE history (see pages 45–46)

➤ when the cough started; production of sputum; thickness and color of sputum; blood in sputum

➤ shortness of breath—constant or only on exertion; difficulty breathing in, breathing out, or both

➤ symptoms of infection (chills, fever, cough, shortness of breath, sore throat, earache, stuffy head)

➤ changes in body temperature, pulse, breathing rate, and skin, lip, and nailbed color

➤ problems in the neck and chest: swollen glands under the jaw, tenderness over or between the ribs, differences in expansion on breathing between one side of the chest and the other. Listen for cough and sounds of abnormal breathing

Consider a respiratory problem serious when

• pain is made worse by coughing or deep breathing, and is accompanied by fever and chills with yellow or green sputum

• there is shortness of breath, weakness, cyanosis, or cold, clammy skin

- the victim is so short of breath he or she cannot speak more than a few words at a time
- it occurs in a person with a history of lung disease, with previous attacks of similar pain
- there is difficulty either in taking air in or blowing it out, accompanied by wheezing, grunting, or snoring
- there is blood in the sputum
- difficulty with inspiration may be accompanied by a crowing sound—*stridor*
- there is known heart disease, pain suggesting a heart attack, an abnormal heart rate (see page 154) or rhythm, and/or marked ankle swelling
- persistent cyanosis of skin, lips, and nailbeds
- shortness of breath of uncertain cause that does not respond to rest or other simple measures

What to Do

If you suspect a serious respiratory problem:

1. Shelter the victim and keep the person warm.
2. Have the person adopt a position that allows the most comfortable breathing.
3. If pain is prominent, give nonprescription pain medication.
4. Give nothing but water or clear, bland liquids by mouth.
5. Arrange immediate evacuation.

For a nonurgent problem:

1. For chest wall pain,
   - Give acetaminophen or ibuprofen and local heat (a washcloth soaked in hot water in a plastic bag—test it on your own skin to be sure it doesn't burn).
   - Lighten the person's load.
2. If the person is short of breath due to an obvious illness, or is markedly more short of breath than his or her companions, move the person to shelter and allow to rest.
3. At altitudes greater than 7,000 feet (2,100 meters), regard significant shortness of breath that does not improve after a few hours rest as altitude sickness; treat by descent (at least 2,000 feet lower;

see page 225). Under no circumstances go any higher unless you have to climb to start the descent.

4. For potentially treatable causes, treat as follows:
    • for nasal congestion: Give nonprescription antihistamine/decongestants according to the package directions.
    • for stridor: If the victim is a child, place the child in a tent with a pan of water boiling on a small stove. *Caution: Be sure the tent is adequately ventilated to avoid risk of fire and carbon monoxide poisoning.* If the victim is an adult, consider allergic swelling of the larynx and give an epinephrine injection if available (see page 205).

5. Evacuate all victims with serious chest problems.

ASTHMA

Asthma is a lung condition with recurring spells of shortness of breath, wheezing, and cough due to spasm and swelling of the small air passages. Attacks result from allergies (to pollen, dust, and animal dander); irritants such as smoke, air pollution, and cold air; or exercise. Asthmatics may be perfectly healthy otherwise and able to participate in strenuous, outdoor activities, especially if the asthma is controlled by medication.

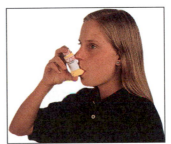

Use of inhaler for asthma attack

What to Look For

Symptoms range from mild to severe and life-threatening.

➤ shortness of breath with difficulty in breathing out; audible wheezing

➤ previous history of asthma

What to Do

1. Place the victim in a comfortable, upright position to help breathing.

2. Assist the person in using medicines as directed on the labels or by the ill person. Most asthmatics carry prescribed medicines (inhaler and/or pills) and know how to use them.

3. Give clear fluids.

4. Evacuate if
- no improvement within 2 hours after using medications
- there are repeated attacks
- there is a severe and prolonged attack
- there is no history of asthma and/or no asthma medicines available

BENIGN HYPERVENTILATION

Many people react to anxiety by overbreathing, or hyperventilating. Hyperventilation by itself, regardless of the cause, can produce alarming symptoms because carbon dioxide is removed from the blood too quickly. This causes

- dizziness or lightheadedness
- increasing shortness of breath
- numbness, coldness, and/or tingling of the mouth, hands, and feet
- blue hands and feet
- sharp or stabbing chest pain

The victim—who believes that these are signs of a heart attack, stroke, or other serious problem—becomes even more anxious, causing more overbreathing that eventually leads to spasmodic contractures of the hands and feet, and fainting. Fainting allows return of normal breathing with recovery.

In the injured and elderly, and those with diabetes, heart disease, or lung disease, always consider serious causes of hyperventilation.

What to Do

If you believe that the hyperventilation is not due to a serious condition:

1. Reassure the person, removing him or her from the cause of anxiety (e.g., a cliff).

2. Encourage slow, regular breathing.

3. If the hyperventilation persists without a precipitating cause, consider other respiratory problems and plan to evacuate.

 DO NOT
- **have the person breathe into a bag since it can dangerously stress the heart and respiratory system.**

Neurologic Emergencies

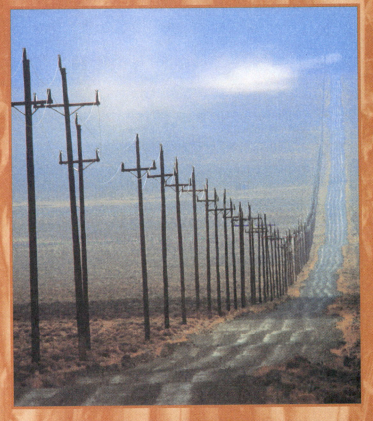

Anatomy and Physiology • The Unresponsive Victim •

The Responsive Victim • Head Injury •

Other Neurologic Problems

Anatomy and Physiology

The nervous system consists of three interconnected parts: the brain, the spinal cord, and the peripheral nerves.

The brain is composed of soft nerve tissue suspended in cerebrospinal fluid, which cushions movement within the rigid, protective skull. The blood supply comes from arteries that run up both sides of the neck and enter the skull from below, then form a delicate network over the surface of the brain. Swelling or bleeding into or around the brain increases pressure within the skull and compresses the brain, compromising cerebral function.

The brain is the "command and control" center of the nervous system, controlling thought and emotion as well as vital bodily functions. The rest of the nervous system is a collection of message lines, conveying signals to and from the brain.

The spinal cord, composed of nerve fibers from the brain, extends from the base of the skull to the lower back. It lies in the spinal canal, protected by the bones of the vertebral column. The peripheral nerves, which arise from the cord and leave the spinal canal between each vertebral bone, carry motor and sensory signals to and from the muscles, skin, and organs of the body.

An injury to the spinal cord affects all functions below the level of the damage.

Brain

Spinal cord

Lies within spinal canal

Peripheral nerves outside spinal canal

Parts of the nervous system

The Unresponsive Victim

An unresponsive victim presents one of the most difficult problems in the wilderness. Regardless of the cause, the first aid management is much the same.

If the victim was observed falling, a traumatic head injury is the likely cause. If there are no witnesses, and the victim is unresponsive, determining the cause may be impossible. Remember that the person may have injured the head from another cause.

If the victim is with another person or group, find out what you can about the person's history. Has the person had a head injury—e.g., from a fall? been unresponsive? had seizures in the past? suffered any known neurologic or other disease? taken any medications or drugs—medicinal or illegal? eaten anything unusual? suffered allergies to food, insect bite, etc.?

Survey the scene to look for clues to the cause if history is unobtainable. Consider the time of year and environment, (e.g., winter—hypothermia; summer—heatstroke). Look for evidence of a fall, boating accident, etc.

What to Look For

Signs of injury include:

➤ blood in the hair

➤ lacerations of the scalp

➤ hematoma (swelling of scalp from bruise with bleeding under the skin)

➤ clear cerebrospinal fluid or blood running from nose or ears

➤ bruising on face

If there is no evidence of injury, assess for:

➤ signs of shock—weak, rapid pulse; pale or cyanotic (blue) skin color

➤ breathing difficulty—rapid, shallow, labored, obstructed

➤ seizure signs—bitten tongue, incontinence of urine, muscle spasms

➤ eyes—turned to one side? pupils equal?

➤ body movements—do both sides of the body move? are movements purposeful or wild, erratic, repetitive?

➤ a response to painful stimuli

➤ medical-alert bracelet or medallion

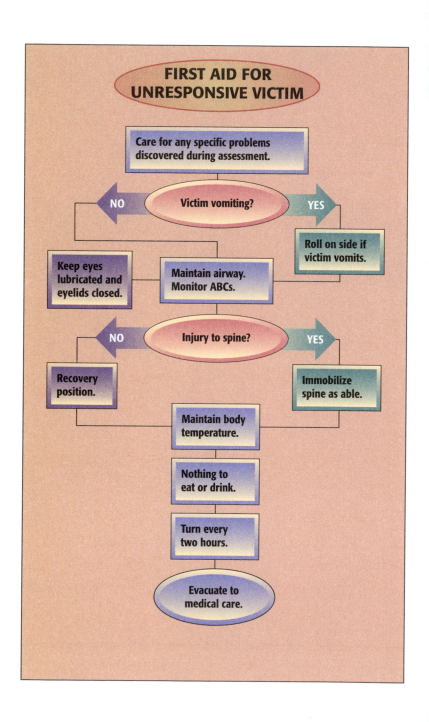

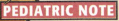

PEDIATRIC NOTE   Closed head injuries are common in children. Direct injury with brain swelling may result in permanent damage. Failure to recognize an inadequate airway can produce a secondary brain injury in children due to lack of oxygen. A child's alertness is a sensitive gauge of adequate oxygenation.

Some Causes of Altered Responsiveness

Head injury
Shock
   heart failure
   severe injury
   bleeding
   spinal injury
Drugs or poisoning
   alcohol
   legal or illegal drugs
   wild plants or mushrooms
Neurologic illness
   stroke
   meningitis
   seizure
Asphyxia
   avalanche burial
   near-drowning
Metabolic and environmental
   low blood sugar
   diabetic coma
   hypothermia
   heatstroke

What to Do

Unresponsiveness has many causes, but all unresponsive or poorly responsive victims need an open airway, protection from aspiration (inhaling into lungs) of saliva and vomit, and a steady, normal body temperature. The general care of all unresponsive victims is similar, regardless of the cause.

With evidence of head injury:

1. Protect the spine in case of fracture or cord injury.
2. Roll the victim carefully onto the back for better examination.
3. . Check ABCs; open and maintain airway.
4. Stop bleeding from scalp wound.
5. Monitor vital signs: one member of party should be with victim at all times.
6. Move victim to safety, comfort, and shelter.
7. Evacuate as soon as possible. Be prepared for vomiting during transportation (see page 170).

Turn an unresponsive, breathing victim without a spine injury to the recovery position.

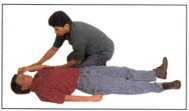

1. Kneel at the victim's side, bend victim's near arm to right angle.

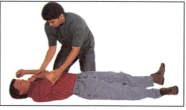

2. Place back of victim's hand against his/her cheek and hold there.

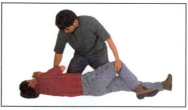

3. Bend victim's far knee. Roll victim toward you so that victim's cheek is on his/her hand.

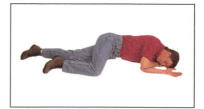

4. Front view of recovery position.

Without evidence of injury (including spinal injury):

1. Roll victim onto back.
2. Check ABCs; open and maintain airway.
3. Turn victim into recovery position when stable.
4. Monitor vital signs.
5. Evacuate as soon as possible.

Evacuate all unresponsive victims rapidly to medical care unless the condition is benign (e.g., simple fainting, page 180), can be treated effectively and rapidly (insulin shock, chapter 13), and is temporary (e.g., epileptic seizure, page 178).

LONG-TERM CARE OF THE UNRESPONSIVE VICTIM

You may have to care for an unresponsive victim for a day or more. If this is the case, avoid pain medications as they may conceal neurologic changes. To encourage emptying a full bladder, stroke the inside of the victim's thigh and pour water loudly from one cup to another. Do not give food or fluid to an unresponsive victim. However, if the victim is unable to take fluids over several days, the person may become seriously dehydrated. Lubricate the eyes with any eye ointment to prevent the cornea from developing ulcers from dry air exposure. Tape the eyelids lightly shut during transportation. Finally, prevent bedsores by turning the victim every 2 hours, and by using scrupulous bowel hygiene to prevent soiling by feces.

The Responsive Victim
What to Look For

Obtain a careful history from the responsive victim or a witness:

➤ details of the accident: exact time, length of fall, etc.

➤ duration of unconsciousness, if any

➤ alterations in behavior or level of consciousness

➤ convulsions

➤ potential for hypothermia at the site of the accident

➤ any known diseases

➤ medical-alert bracelet or medallion, which may tell of known illnesses (epilepsy, diabetes, heart attack) that might have caused the loss of consciousness instead of the head injury

➤ smell of alcohol on the breath or the sweet smell of diabetes

➤ level of consciousness: use the AVPU scale to measure. Restlessness may be due to brain injury or pain.

➤ unequal pupil size, indicating possible damage to one side of the brain

➤ spinal injury: may occur with the head injury

➤ blood or clear fluid oozing or dripping from the nose or ears, without a local injury to account for it, which may suggest bleeding or leaking of cerebrospinal fluid from a fracture of the base of the skull

Head Injury

People with serious head injuries tend to get worse and die; those with less severe head injuries tend to get better. Very few head injuries need surgery; those that do need it at once.

TYPES OF HEAD INJURY

Injuries to the head may involve the brain, the soft tissues of the scalp, or the bony skull. Three main types of injury may occur.

Concussion   Even a mild blow on the head can jar the brain against the skull and momentarily disrupt mental function. Anyone who has been unresponsive from a head injury, however briefly, must not walk or be left unattended because intracranial bleeding may occur during the next few hours, resulting in disorientation or even coma.

What to Look For

➤ A person who falls unconscious briefly may "see stars."

➤ After rest, recovery may be quick and complete.

➤ Recent memory is affected (amnesia for the injury event), and the person may ask the same question repeatedly.

What to Do

1. Following a concussion, allow the victim to sleep, but wake the person every 2–3 hours to check level of responsiveness.

2. If no symptoms appear 8 hours after injury, wake once during the first night.

Bruising or Hemorrhage with Delayed Deterioration   More severe injury may bruise the brain or rupture blood vessels. The resulting swelling or bleeding causes increased pressure inside the skull, which interferes with brain function. The victim will die unless the blood under pressure is released quickly by surgery. Brain damage from compression may be permanent because brain cells cannot regenerate (unlike cells in other parts of the body).

What to Look For

➤ After a head injury the victim may regain consciousness, appear quite normal (lucid interval), and continue the expedition. However, continued bleeding or swelling of the brain causes pressure inside the skull to rise.

➤ victim complaints of severe, progressive headache not relieved by common medications

➤ repeated vomiting

➤ altered behavior: confusion, combativeness, irrationality, or apparent intoxication; then drowsiness and progressive unresponsiveness

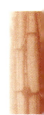

What to Do

1. Protect and maintain the airway.
2. Maintain a stable body temperature.
3. Treat as though unresponsive (see page 169).
4. Evacuate immediately.

Severe, Diffuse Injury   Severe, diffuse injury with unresponsiveness from time of injury may be caused either by the initial injury to the brain and subsequent swelling, or by lack of oxygen (hypoxia) secondary to inadequate breathing (asphyxia) or drowning.

What to Look For

➤ The victim is deeply unconscious from the time of injury.

➤ The airway may be obstructed and breathing impaired.

➤ Re-evaluate frequently according to the AVPU scale (see page 48). Changes in responsiveness over time are extremely important. Improvement is a good sign, deterioration is ominous.

➤ Monitor the speed of regaining normal consciousness; this indicates roughly the severity of the injury and forecasts the final outcome.

Good Signs

• Victim starts to awaken, responds verbally, knows his or her name, whereabouts, month, and year.

- Body movements become normal and are equal on both sides.
- Victim blinks in response to a close hand wave.

Bad Signs

- Pupils fail to respond to light.
- One pupil becomes larger than the other.
- Pulse slows.
- Breathing becomes irregular.
- Temperature rises.
- Victim awakens but there is evidence of brain or spinal damage with loss of feeling, one-sided weakness, or paralysis.

What to Do

1. Clear and maintain the airway; if no respirations, start rescue breathing.
2. Assume spinal cord injuries.
3. Apply a neck collar, or otherwise restrain the head from moving (see page 54).
4. Repeat examination periodically to determine progress; record observations.
5. Prevent additional injury: move the victim to shelter and safety.
6. Evacuate quickly.
7. For care of the responsive victim, see chapter 3.
8. For care of the unresponsive victim, see chapter 3.

SKULL FRACTURES

Fractures may be "closed" or "open." A *closed* fracture occurs without a break in the scalp. A fracture is *open* when the bony skull is breached and the brain or its coverings exposed. Skull fractures may occur without displacement of bone, or with a depressed segment of bone that may press on the brain.

What to Look For

➤ broken bone edges in the wound (A smooth exposed white bone surface may not be serious if there is no associated skull fracture.)

➤ fracture at base of skull—clear or blood-tinged fluid dripping from the nose or ear without apparent injury to account for it

What to Do

1. Press around the wound edge on undamaged skull using a dough-nut dressing so nothing disturbs the fracture.

2. If there is an open fracture, cover the wound with a sterile dressing.

3. Evacuate.

Other Neurologic Problems
STROKE

Stroke is caused by blockage of a blood vessel or bleeding in the brain. If an artery is partially blocked, the stroke symptoms may be temporary. These "little strokes," known as transient ischemic attacks (TIAs), last from a few minutes to several hours, after which the victim recovers.

Stroke is most common in those with "hardening of the arteries" (arteriosclerosis), the elderly, and those with high blood pressure or diabetes. In the wilderness, symptoms of stroke occasionally occur in young, healthy persons due to a head injury, decompression sickness, or cerebral edema (HACE, see pages 227–229) or thickening of the blood due to altitude.

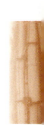

What to Look For

The signs and symptoms of stroke depend on the part of the brain involved.

➤ altered responsiveness: assess as for unresponsive victim (see page 169)

➤ numbness, weakness, or paralysis of face, arm, or leg, usually on one side of the body

➤ turning of the head and eyes to one side

➤ noisy breathing, drooling

➤ visual changes: double vision; sudden blurring or loss of vision in one or both eyes

➤ loss of balance or coordination

➤ difficulty speaking or inability to understand simple statements

➤ sudden, very severe, unexplained, long-lasting headache

➤ convulsions

➤ a history of diabetes, hypertension, heart disease, or previous strokes

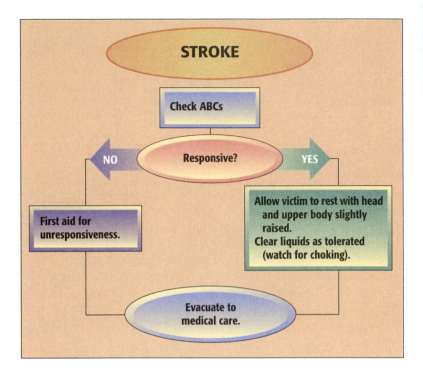

What to Do

1. Keep victim in recovery position (see page 41), with head and upper body slightly raised to lessen brain swelling.

2. If victim is awake, allow the person to find a comfortable position.

3. Offer clear liquids with caution.

4. Evacuate.

SEIZURES

Seizures are due to sudden, temporary, abnormal electrical discharges in the brain. Recurrent seizures occur in epilepsy.

There are two types of seizures. *Partial* seizures are a momentary lack of awareness, an involuntary movement of an arm, leg, and/or face, a sensation of numbness or tingling, or abnormal vision or smell. Consciousness may or may not be affected. *Generalized* seizures are frequently preceded by an "aura"—a momentary vision, smell, or other sensation that forewarns the victim of the seizure—then start with a sudden spasm of body muscles, causing the victim to cry out hoarsely and fall to the ground with rigid back and limbs. A few seconds later, violent, rhythmic contractions of the neck, back, and extremities occur. During this phase, which usually lasts only a few minutes, the victim may bite the tongue or be incontinent. After a seizure, the victim is unresponsive for minutes to an hour or longer, then gradually awakens. Immediately after a seizure, the victim breathes deeply, may look blue, and "foam at the mouth."

In people with known epilepsy, seizures are rarely medical emergencies. They end after a few minutes and aren't associated with harm unless the victim is in a dangerous or exposed location or is injured during the seizure. The victim usually does not require medical attention.

Most epileptics can control their seizures with medication and live a normal life, including participating in wilderness activities. However, they should avoid dangerous activities (climbing, alpine skiing, riding chair-lifts, unsupervised swimming, boating, scuba diving, and caving) unless they have a history of reliably taking medicine on schedule, have been seizure-free for at least two years, and have permission from their neurologist.

Causes of Seizures in People without Known Epilepsy

Head injury	Stroke
Hypoglycemia	Lightning injury
Poisoning	Illegal drugs
Heatstroke	Oxygen lack
High fever (children)	Pregnancy (toxemia)

What to Do

1. An oncoming seizure cannot be prevented. Concentrate on preventing injury. Help the victim to lie down in a safe area.

2. Don't restrain the victim. If possible, remove nearby objects that the victim might strike. Don't open or insert anything into victim's mouth.

3. Breathing may stop temporarily, but will restart *without* help. After the seizure make sure the airway is open.

4. The victim may have been incontinent and may be embarrassed; discourage onlookers and arrange for privacy.

5. Afterward, the victim will have an altered mental status or be sleepy. Assess as you would for the unresponsive victim (see page 169). In particular, take the body temperature (heatstroke) if you have a thermometer, feel the skin temperature, and look for lacerations of the tongue or injuries caused by muscle spasms or a fall. Look for a medical-alert tag. Keep the victim in the recovery position (see page 41) until awake and alert.

6. Check for a history of seizures. If so, is medicine being taken to prevent seizures? Have any doses been missed?

7. If there is no history of epilepsy, ask about diabetes, a recent head injury, eating wild plants, and medicines or illegal drugs taken. If the victim is a child, ask the parents whether he or she has had a high fever.

8. Evacuate if
   • no history of epilepsy with similar episodes
   • the seizure lasts more than 5 minutes or seizures are repetitive
   • responsiveness does not return within 2 hours
   • victim is in last half of pregnancy

Common Medicines for Epilepsy that Victim Might Be Carrying

Dilantin	Phenobarbital
Tegretol	Mysoline
Depakene	Zarontin
Tridione	

SIMPLE FAINTING

Simple fainting is a common, benign, and usually brief form of rapid drop in blood pressure that results in inadequate blood flow to the brain and loss of normal responsiveness. It may have either a physical or an emotional cause: pain, the sight of blood, excitement, fear, or standing for a long time, especially in the heat. Someone who is dehydrated or has lost blood may faint on trying to stand.

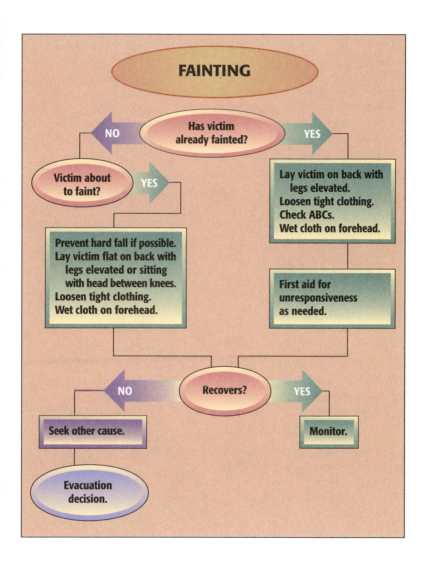

What to Look For

In a previously healthy person:

➤ reports of "seeing spots," feeling dizzy, hot or cold, and nauseated

➤ paleness, with cold, clammy skin

➤ "passing out," and slumping or falling down

What to Do

For a person about to faint:

1. Prevent a hard, injury-causing fall.

2. Lay the person flat immediately. Raise the legs 8–12 inches. If there is no place to lie down, the person should sit with the head between the knees. (When the person is flat on the ground, blood flow to the brain increases, blood pressure returns rapidly to normal, and the victim wakes up.)

3. Loosen tight clothing, especially around the neck.

4. Place a cool, wet cloth on the forehead.

If the person has fainted:

1. Check the ABCs.

2. Lay the victim flat and raise the legs 8–12 inches.

3. Loosen tight clothing.

4. Check for injuries caused by the fall.

5. Place a cool, wet cloth on forehead.

6. Provide care for unresponsiveness (see "The Unresponsive Victim," page 169).

7. Keep the person lying down until he or she has recovered, then have the victim stand up slowly.

8. Evacuate, if the victim
   • appears to have a serious illness or injury
   • has fainted repeatedly
   • does not awaken within 30 minutes
   • was lying down when the episode occurred
   • continues to be lightheaded when attempting to get up

Unresponsiveness due to a sudden serious illness (heart attack, stroke, internal bleeding with shock) may be mistaken at first for a simple faint. A middle-aged or elderly victim, or one who doesn't recover rapidly after lying flat, should be assessed and cared for as any unresponsive victim. If fainting occurs each time the person stands, suspect internal bleeding.

HEADACHE

Most headaches are harmless and can be controlled by resting, avoiding eye fatigue, and by taking mild, nonprescription medications (aspirin, acetaminophen, or ibuprofen). In the wilderness, headaches can also be caused by altitude, glare off snow or water, and traction on the neck muscles from carrying a heavy pack.

Rarely, a headache may be the first sign of a serious condition, such as HACE (see pages 227–229), stroke, meningitis, or severe high blood pressure.

What to Look For

➤ head trauma

➤ tenderness over the scalp, neck, and shoulders due to chronic muscle contraction

➤ pupils unequal in size

➤ complaints of double vision (stroke)

➤ fever

➤ severe neck stiffness

➤ impaired sensation or movement of the extremities (stroke)

➤ impaired balance: have the victim stand with the eyes closed or walk a straight line (test for HACE)

Suspect serious illness or injury if headache:

➤ causes vomiting, inability to sleep, or inability to eat or drink for more than a day in someone *without* previous recurrent headaches (even if infrequent)

➤ lasts more than a day, is unresponsive to nonprescription medication, and is steadily getting worse

➤ is sudden and severe, unlike any previous headaches, and does not improve with rest and mild pain medicine

➤ is associated with drowsiness, stiff neck, altered mental status, high fever, personality changes, visual changes, weakness or loss of sensation on one side of the body, and/or loss of balance

What to Do

1. If headache is mild to moderate, give nonprescription pain medication.

2. If acute mountain sickness (see pages 224–229) is a possibility, descend to an altitude below that at which the headache started (at least 2,000 feet lower). Do **not** go higher!

3. If the cause appears serious, evacuate.

MIGRAINE

Migraine headaches are usually periodic, one-sided, throbbing, and frequently accompanied by nausea and vomiting. They tend to run in families and affect men less frequently than women, in whom they may occur around the time of the menstrual period. The headaches are frequently preceded by a warning "aura" (spots or bright lights). Migraine sufferers usually carry medication to be taken at the onset of a headache; if not, sometimes mild nonprescription pain medications help. During the headache, allow the victim to rest in a dark area.

DIABETES (SEE CHAPTER 13)

Diabetics are subject to alterations in blood sugar that affect their responsiveness.

Low blood sugar (hypoglycemia) can be caused by taking too much insulin, or by taking insulin but not enough food. Exercise lowers blood sugar and diabetics not used to strenuous hiking or other exercise may not eat enough extra food to prevent a significant drop in blood sugar. Hypoglycemic fainting comes on quickly, with dizziness, sweating and alteration of responsiveness. Treat by giving sugar immediately. Recovery is usually rapid.

High blood sugar levels (hyperglycemia) result from too little insulin. Blood sugar levels climb slowly, sometimes over a day or two. The condition is recognized by excessive thirst, large urine output, exhaustion, or a "fruity" smell to the breath. As the condition worsens the person may lapse into coma. This is very dangerous and requires evacuation.

CHAPTER 12

Abdominal Emergencies

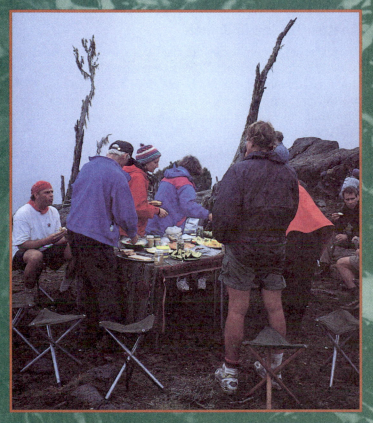

Anatomy of the Abdomen • Injuries • Illnesses •

Bloody Stools and Hemorrhoids • Hernia •

Evacuation Guidelines for Abdominal Problems

Abdominal problems are difficult to diagnose even in a hospital, and a first-aider should not be expected to distinguish among the many causes of abdominal pain; usually, first aid will be similar regardless of the cause. For wilderness first aid, it is most useful to consider abdominal problems according to the few common symptoms they cause rather than offer a diagnosis. A few common specific problems are discussed. The major decision in the wilderness is when to evacuate the victim.

Anatomy of the Abdomen

The abdomen is bounded by the diaphragm above and the bony pelvis below. Within the cavity of the abdomen lie the liver, kidneys, spleen, stomach, and the small and large intestines. The intestines (somewhat like the lungs) are enclosed in a membrane, the *peritoneum*, and are surrounded by the peritoneal space or cavity in which blood or other fluids can collect. The aorta and inferior vena cava, the two largest blood vessels in the body, run along the back wall of the abdomen against the vertebral column.

Anterior means that the organs lie toward the front; *posterior* means that they lie against the back wall of the abdominal cavity. When communicating to potential rescuers or considering certain problems, divide the abdomen into four quadrants. Pain localized in one of these areas may indicate a particular problem. For example, pain with soreness to pressure in the right upper quadrant may be from a liver injury or infection (hepatitis), or the gallbladder blocked by a stone; pain in

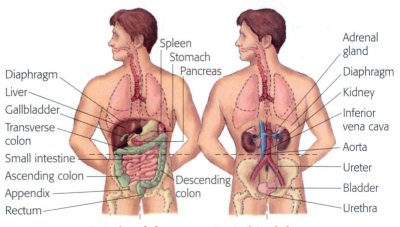

Anterior abdomen   **Posterior abdomen**

Anatomy and contents of the abdomen

the right lower quadrant may be from appendicitis, an ovarian or pregnancy problem, kidney stone, or hernia on that side; left lower quadrant pain may be from a problem in the bowel, ovary, kidney stone, or hernia on that side; and left upper quadrant pain may be from an injury to the spleen, stomach, or pancreas.

Pain in both front and back often points to one of the organs in the posterior abdomen. When on one side, the problem may be in the kidney (infection or stone), gallbladder (on the right), or a major blood vessel. When in the midline, it may be from the pancreas, stomach, aorta, or uterus. Injuries to intra-abdominal organs can be categorized as *closed* (resulting from falls and blows) or *open* (resulting from penetration by knife, stick, rock, bullet, etc.). Illnesses include diarrheal diseases (e.g., gastroenteritis), pain of unknown origin, bleeding, intestinal blockage, and hernia.

Injuries

Serious injury to the abdomen, whether blunt, without a break in the skin (closed), or with penetration of the peritoneal cavity (open), may cause internal bleeding or leakage of intestinal contents that cause irritation and infection (peritonitis) within the peritoneal cavity. Surgery is the treatment for most serious internal abdominal injuries. Look for an associated abdominal injury with injuries of the lower chest.

CLOSED INJURIES
What to Look For

➤ mechanism of injury

➤ bruising or abrasions of abdominal wall or lower chest

➤ abdominal pain and tenderness of varying severity. If severe, the person lies quite still. Pain usually starts around the navel, then spreads to the region of the injured organ. If blood or intestinal contents are in the abdominal cavity, pain may be felt in one or both shoulders.

➤ signs of shock (see page 150)

➤ the combination of an enlarged tight abdomen, increasing pain and tenderness, fever, and nausea and vomiting—highly suspicious signs of peritonitis, due either to injury or illness. The abdomen becomes more rigid as peritonitis spreads; movement, coughing, and tapping or pressing on the abdomen causes pain.

> nausea and vomiting
> external bleeding from a laceration of the abdominal wall

What to Do

1. Rest the victim completely and allow only sips of water by mouth.

2. Record written observations frequently, especially the pulse rate and changes in general condition.

3. Evacuate if any signs of shock or peritonitis appear.

OPEN INJURIES

An abdominal injury is "open" if there is more than a superficial injury to the skin, with or without obvious penetration of the peritoneal cavity.

What to Look For

> A small puncture wound of the abdominal skin can be as dangerous as an obvious gash. A long, sharp object that punctures the skin can be withdrawn, leaving barely a mark; but a punctured bowel may seal over temporarily and leak intestinal contents later.

> protruding bowel or fat

What to Do

If the object that caused the injury is still in the wound, and if medical help is close by, leave the object there—as taught in urban first aid. If the object has penetrated one of the large blood vessels but is blocking the escape of blood, severe bleeding might occur with removal. Otherwise, no additional harm will come from removing it, even if the object has penetrated the peritoneal cavity and the intestine. So, if medical help is a long distance away and the victim needs to be transported over rough terrain with the risk of moving the object despite bandage stabilization, remove the object.

1. Treat as for closed injuries.

2. If bowel is protruding and has not been torn, two options are available. If help is far away, try to return the bowel gently to the abdominal cavity; then dress the wound. If help is close at hand, cover the bowel with a moist (preferably sterile) cloth. Keep the wound moist during transportation.

3. If the bowel has been torn it must *not* be returned to the abdominal cavity. Cover it and keep it moist.

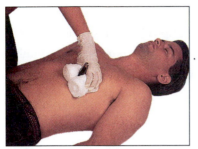

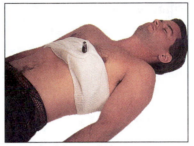

Stabilize penetrating object with bulky padding.

Secure padding and object.

SPECIFIC INJURIES

Evacuate all victims with the following injuries.

Spleen   A blow to the left upper abdomen or fractured lower left ribs can rupture the spleen. Consider splenic rupture after a lower left chest injury. Shock, due to progressive severe bleeding, develops after rupture. Silent symptomless bleeding may continue from several hours to 3 weeks beneath the capsule of the spleen until it suddenly bursts, resulting in immediate shock.

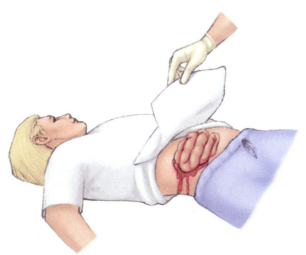

Open wound with protruding bowel

What to Look For

➤ pain in the left flank or over the left upper part of the abdomen

➤ immediate, severe shock caused by bleeding into the peritoneum

Liver   Injury may be caused by a crushing blow to the upper abdomen or by fracture of the right lower ribs.

What to Look For

➤ signs of shock

➤ pain in the right upper abdomen

Kidney   Injury may be caused by a direct blow to the back or flank, possibly with a fracture of the lowest rib.

What to Look For

➤ pain in the flank, sometimes radiating down into the groin

➤ blood in the urine

PEDIATRIC NOTE   The abdominal contents are less well protected in a child than in an adult. The rib cage does not cover the liver or spleen, and the pelvis is relatively shallow, allowing greater exposure to injury.

Illnesses

PAIN

Do not attempt to determine the cause of pain but decide when to evacuate the victim, with or without help. This decision is sometimes immediately apparent, but you may have to observe the victim for several hours to determine the course of the illness. (See the criteria for evacuation at the end of this chapter.) The difficulty in obtaining help, the number of people in the group (can the person be left alone while you go for help?), and other factors affect this decision.

What to Look For (All Causes)

➤ signs of shock, caused by internal bleeding or infection

➤ a SAMPLE history (see pages 45–46)

➤ Where is the pain? The cause of the pain may be in the organ underlying the site.

➤ Is the pain decreasing, increasing, or staying the same?

➤ Is there associated diarrhea or vomiting?

➤ If there has been repeated vomiting and or diarrhea, are there signs of dehydration—dry tongue, rapid pulse, dizziness on standing?

➤ Does anyone else in the party have the same problem?

➤ Are there associated conditions such as diabetes or pregnancy?

➤ Is the abdomen painful, rigid, or abnormally swollen?

Note: See chapter 14 regarding low abdominal pain in females and the management of kidney stones.

What to Do

1. Make an initial check and assess vital signs (see chapter 3).

2. Allow slow sipping of clear fluids: water, diluted juice, sports drinks, soup broth, herbal tea. (Avoid alcohol or caffeine-containing drinks.) (See appendix D for fluid and electrolyte replacement guidelines.)

3. Give an antacid.

4. Apply heat, such as a canteen filled with warm water, to the abdomen.

5. Be prepared for vomiting.

6. Allow victim to assume the most comfortable position, often lying with knees bent.

DO NOT
- **give an enema or laxative. These may worsen the condition or cause complications.**
- **give nonclear fluids to drink as long as the pain continues.**
- **give solid foods.**
- **give milk products.**

APPENDICITIS
What to Look For

➤ Intermittent pain that begins in the midabdomen, then moves to the lower right abdomen. The pain increases over 6 to 24 hours, becomes constant, and is accentuated by movement or cough, causing the victim to lie still with the knees drawn up

➤ tenderness to pressure or touch over the lower right abdomen

➤ intermittent vomiting

➤ diarrhea (possible but not usual)

➤ loss of appetite

➤ low-grade fever

➤ pain and tenderness felt throughout the abdomen, indicating a ruptured appendix, spreading infection throughout the abdominal cavity (peritonitis)

What to Do

1. Place the victim in the most comfortable reclining position.
2. Give sips of fluid to avoid dehydration, but avoid food.
3. Evacuate.

NAUSEA AND VOMITING

Nausea and vomiting may occur with many conditions such as mild altitude sickness, motion sickness, head injury, intestinal viruses, food poisoning, excessive eating or drinking, carbon monoxide poisoning, or emotional stress. In minor illnesses, this should improve within a couple of days. Persistent or increasing nausea and vomiting may signal more serious illnesses such as appendicitis or bowel obstruction. If the condition lasts longer than 1 or 2 days, serious dehydration may develop, especially in young children and the elderly.

What to Look For

➤ abdominal pain

➤ blood or brown, grainy material (looks like coffee grounds) in the vomit; this could be blood from the stomach

➤ diarrhea; vomiting and diarrhea together are often a self-limited viral infection

➤ chills and fever

➤ signs of dehydration (i.e., dizziness when standing, dry mouth and tongue, cracked lips, thirst, rapid pulse)

➤ others in the group with similar symptoms (suggests food poisoning or infectious cause)

➤ recent head injury (see chapter 6)

➤ wild mushroom/plant ingestion

What to Do

1. Give small amounts of clear fluids—sports drinks, clear soups, flat soda, apple or cranberry juice (see appendix D for fluid and electrolyte replacement guidelines).

2. If victim is able to keep fluids down, offer carbohydrates (starches, bread, cereal, and pasta) first—these are the easiest to digest. Avoid any milk products or meats for 48 hours.

3. Have the victim rest—avoid exertion until he or she is able to eat solid foods easily.

DIARRHEA

Diarrhea is the frequent passage of loose, watery, or unformed stools. Common causes are intestinal infections (bacterial, viral, or parasitic), food poisoning, food sensitivity/allergy, and stress. Dehydration occurs if the victim cannot drink enough fluid to replace the losses from diarrhea. The elderly and very young are especially prone to dehydration. Replacement of fluids and electrolytes (sodium and potassium) is of primary importance in any diarrhea victim.

What to Look For

➤ bloody mucus or pus in the stool

➤ signs of dehydration

➤ cramping abdominal pain, usually in the lower abdomen

➤ lack of bowel control

➤ fever

➤ others in the group with similar symptoms

What to Do

1. Have the victim drink enough clear fluids to replace losses plus the usual intake. Watch urine output to gauge adequacy of fluid intake. Scant dark urine indicates dehydration.

2. When clear fluids are tolerated, have the victim return gradually to a normal diet. Try crackers, soup, toast, rice, pasta, applesauce.

3. If available, give Pepto-Bismol™ (adult dose: 2 tabs 4 times per day for 1 or 2 days or 2 tablespoons every ½ hour for 8 doses).

4. Give Imodium A-D™ (capsule or liquid, 2–4 mg initially, then 1–2 mg 4 times a day if diarrhea persists) or Lomotil™ (prescription drug). Do not use if there are fever and diarrhea with blood or pus in the stools.

Avoid

➤ milk products or meats for 48 hours after diarrhea stops because there may be intolerance to fat or lactose after infections

➤ caffeine, because it stimulates the intestine and increases urination and dehydration

CONSTIPATION

Minor changes in diet, fluid intake, activity, and emotional state can cause constipation. Changing these will relieve constipation in most cases.

Avoid

➤ strong laxatives, alcohol, and "binding" foods (bananas, cheese, applesauce, and chocolate)

Bloody Stools and Hemorrhoids

Small amounts of bright red blood on the stool and toilet paper or in the toilet water is alarming but usually not serious. More serious bleeding from growths farther inside the rectum is usually darker in color. There are two common causes: hemorrhoids (piles) and fissures. Hemorrhoids are inflamed, swollen veins, and fissures are cracks in the skin around the anus. Both may be caused by constipation with hard, dry stools that require straining to evacuate. Constipation and these resulting problems are common at high altitude or in other environments where it may be impossible to drink enough fluids and eat enough fruit, vegetables, and fiber. Hemorrhoids may also occur with frequent diarrheal bowel movements. Hemorrhoids and fissures may resolve by themselves, but commonly recur.

What to Look For

External Hemorrhoid

➤ a firm, painful, pink or bluish lump next to the anus present for several days.

➤ bright red blood and small dark clots possibly extruding from the swelling: with bleeding, pain and swelling decrease. The discomfort of external hemorrhoids resolves naturally in about 1 week, with or without bleeding.

Internal Hemorrhoid

➤ soft swelling, often painless, frequently protruding from the rectum during or after a bowel movement; may be internal and invisible

➤ bleeding with passage of stool (either type of hemorrhoid)

Fissure

➤ painful crack in the skin at the margin of the anus

Signs of Serious Bowel Bleeding

➤ painless bowel movements with large quantities of red, maroon, or brownish blood (there may be some abdominal cramping)

➤ signs of shock from blood loss (see page 150)

What to Do

For Minor Hemorrhoids and Fissures with Bleeding

1. Adjust diet to soften stool. Increase fluids, fruits, vegetables, and whole grains.

2. Give warm baths to soothe and cleanse.

3. Have the victim wear cotton underwear and loose clothing.

4. Apply cold compresses, zinc oxide, or petroleum jelly to control irritation.

5. Apply hemorrhoid suppositories to help relieve pain.

6. If a grapelike cluster or large swelling protrudes from the rectum, have the victim get on the knees and elbows with the buttocks higher than the head, and apply gentle steady manual pressure to the protruding tissue until it slips back inside. The person should remain in this position or lie on the side for about 30–60 minutes.

For Major Bleeding

1. Have the victim walk if not dizzy or weak.

2. Evacuate.

Hernia

Hernias occur when loops of intestines protrude through a weak spot in the abdominal wall. This condition is more common in men than women, and the most common site is the groin. Other possible sites are the navel and old surgical scars. Hernias may appear suddenly or enlarge gradually. They rarely require urgent surgery, and most hernias will easily slide back inside (reduce) with relaxation and gentle pressure. Occasionally a hernia is trapped and the blood supply to the protruding loop of intestine is cut off (strangulated hernia). This requires emergency medical care.

What to Look For

Unstrangulated Hernia

➤ bulging in groin, sometimes extending into the scrotum; easier to see when victim is straining or coughing and disappears (reduces) if the person lies on the back and relaxes the abdomen

➤ swelling, usually soft and painless

➤ soreness, burning or feeling of pressure (variable)

Strangulated Hernia

➤ hernia that will not reduce

➤ firm bulge with rapidly increasing pain, tenderness

➤ pain spreading to abdomen; possible vomiting

What to Do

1. The victim may continue activities if there is minimal soreness.

2. For possible strangulated hernia, attempt to reduce by having the victim lie on the back and relax. Apply steady, gentle pressure to push the hernia back through its opening. If reduction is not easy, *do not persist.*

3. Evacuate if there is increasing pain and you are unable to reduce the hernia.

Evacuation Guidelines for Abdominal Problems

Evacuate to medical care if

- the victim has sustained a serious injury
- there is persistent abdominal pain for more than 8 hours
- the person is unable to drink or retain fluids for more than 24 hours
- the victim is a pregnant woman with abdominal pain
- the abdomen is rigid or swollen and painful
- the pain increases with cough or movement
- the victim has persistent pain that begins around the navel and later moves to the lower right abdomen (appendicitis)
- the victim has abdominal pain with high fever
- there is vomiting or diarrhea with severe pain
- there is vomiting with severe headache (and no history of migraine or a recent head injury)
- there are signs of internal bleeding: stool or vomit is bloody, stool appears black (Pepto-Bismol™ causes black/gray stools), or vomitus appears brown and grainy, like coffee grounds
- the victim has diarrhea with fever and stools containing bloody mucus
- there are signs of severe dehydration or shock (see chapter 9): fainting or extreme light-headedness when trying to stand, rapid pulse, altered mental status

Diabetic Emergencies and Allergies

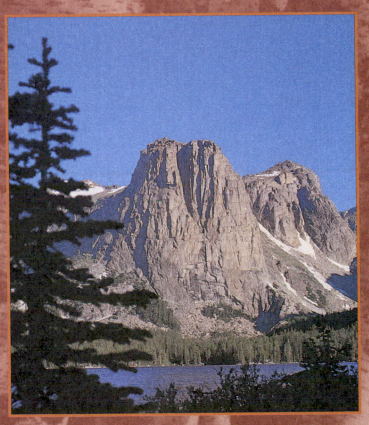

Diabetes • Acute Complications of Diabetes •

Allergic Reactions and Anaphylactic Shock

Glucose, the sugar in the blood, is the basic fuel for most normal metabolic processes. To be able to use glucose, cells require insulin, a hormone produced by the pancreas. In diabetes, insulin is either lacking or ineffective. A wilderness emergency occurs when a diabetic's insulin and blood sugar levels go out of balance.

Diabetes

There are two types of diabetes:

1. *Type I: juvenile-onset (or insulin dependent).* The body produces little or no insulin. The person must take daily insulin injections, regulate calorie intake, and limit sugar and sweets. With good control of the disease, Type I diabetics can live relatively normal lives and participate in wilderness activities. However, if injured or unable to eat properly or take their insulin on schedule, they are likely to become ill within 24 hours.

2. *Type II: adult-onset (frequently not insulin dependent).* Sufferers are older and usually overweight. Their bodies do not produce enough insulin. Although this type of diabetes can frequently be controlled by diet and weight loss, diabetes control medicine (insulin or oral medication to increase insulin production) may also be required. If in good physical condition, these diabetics can participate in strenuous wilderness activities. They are less likely than juvenile onset diabetics to develop acute complications.

DIABETICS IN THE WILDERNESS

All diabetics need to eat on a regular schedule and plan the timing and amount of exercise, since physical exertion acts like insulin. A diabetic who plans to exercise vigorously needs to take less diabetic control medicine or eat more in order to avoid serious drops in blood sugar. If a diabetic's blood sugar levels remain abnormal for long, a wilderness emergency will occur.

Good diabetes management requires frequent measurement of blood glucose levels with a chemically treated paper strip or an electronic blood sugar analyzer.

Before starting on a wilderness trip, diabetics must inform the wilderness group leader that they are diabetic; discuss the planned trip with their physician; and carry adequate supplies of necessary medicines and other equipment (insulin, syringes, needles, pills, etc.), including extra supplies for emergencies. (Another party member might agree to carry these extra supplies.) They should also carry extra food and snacks, so that they do not have to rely on others in the group if food is needed quickly.

Diabetic Supplies

- insulin or diabetes control pills
- syringes, needles, alcohol wipes
- equipment to measure blood sugar
- oral glucose tablets, candy bars, and/or plastic bottles of thick glucose solution ("Glutose")
- injectable medicine to raise low blood sugar (glucagon)

If you are a trip leader with a diabetic group member, refresh your memory regarding diabetic first aid problems; see that at least one other party member is also familiar with these problems; and ideally, if the diabetic takes insulin, ensure that at least one additional party member knows how to give injections.

Insulin and glucagon should be protected from cold (in an inside pocket in cold weather) or heat (in a closed vacuum bottle or buried in the pack). Insulin will not work in hypothermic patients if body temperature is below 30°C (88°F).

Acute Complications of Diabetes
INSULIN SHOCK

Insulin shock occurs if the diabetic is getting too much insulin, too much exercise, or too little food (or a combination of these), which causes the blood sugar level to fall too low (hypoglycemia). Since the brain is very sensitive to lack of sugar, the person rapidly becomes sweaty, faint, dizzy, and may become unresponsive quite rapidly.

KETOACIDOSIS

Ketoacidosis occurs when the diabetic has too little insulin, which allows blood sugar levels to become too high. This causes dehydration, weight loss, increased thirst, and passage of large amounts of urine.

Ketoacidosis develops more slowly than insulin shock but also will progress to an unresponsive state called *diabetic coma*. If not treated, diabetic coma will lead to death within a few hours or days. Ketoacidosis tends to occur in insulin-dependent diabetics who fail to take enough insulin. It also can occur in a diabetic after an injury or with an acute

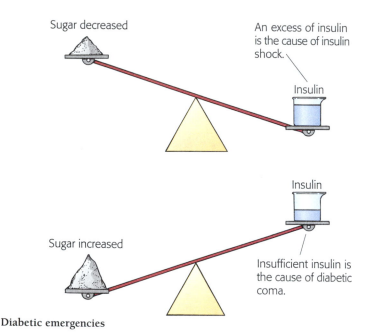

Sugar decreased

An excess of insulin is the cause of insulin shock.

Insulin

Insulin

Sugar increased

Insufficient insulin is the cause of diabetic coma.

Diabetic emergencies

medical condition such as pneumonia or gastroenteritis with nausea and vomiting, because requirements for insulin increase.

What to Look For

Insulin Shock (Blood Sugar Too Low)
➤ sudden onset (minutes to an hour)
➤ pale, cold, clammy skin
➤ rapid pulse
➤ headache, hunger, dizziness, nervousness, weakness
➤ staggering, poor coordination, trembling
➤ personality changes: anger, bad temper
➤ altered mental status (confusion, disorientation, eventual coma)

Ketoacidosis (Blood Sugar Too High)
➤ gradual onset (hours to days)
➤ flushed, dry, warm skin
➤ rapid pulse
➤ rapid, deep respirations

➤ extreme thirst

➤ "fruity" odor of breath

➤ vomiting

➤ frequent urination

➤ altered mental status (drowsiness, confusion, eventual coma)

What to Do

1. Immediately check diabetics whose behavior is unusual.

2. Determine if the victim has an illness or an injury (or both). Is the person responsive or unresponsive? Consider hypoglycemia in young, healthy-appearing people with sudden faintness, sweating, and confusion. **Look for a medical-alert tag**.

3. Do an initial check and care for immediate problems. If victim is unresponsive, assess condition of the head, ability to move, and response to pain.

4. Do an ongoing assessment. Determine what has happened, prior history of diabetes or other medical conditions, and whether the victim has been taking any medicines or shots. Find out when the diabetic ate last, and whether insulin or other diabetic medications were taken that day.

5. In the victim with altered mental status, *as soon as it is discovered that the victim is diabetic*, immediately give sugar (candy, a sugar-containing drink, or several spoonfuls of table sugar preferably dissolved in water) *while he or she can still swallow*. If blood sugar is low, it will rise quickly; if the victim is in ketoacidosis, the extra sugar will do no harm.

6. If the victim is unable to swallow, place a thick glucose solution (if available) or a paste made of water and sugar between the cheek and the gum, where it may be swallowed reflexly.

7. The diabetic with normal mental status may be able to tell you what the problem is. In this case, *if requested*, help the person take sugar or a diabetic control medication—including injections of insulin or glucagon, a substance that raises blood sugar.

8. A diabetic recovering from hypoglycemia after receiving sugar needs a meal and rest before resuming normal activity.

9. Evacuate those who don't recover or become worse. If ketoacidosis is suspected, give nonsugar-containing liquids if the victim can swallow and is not vomiting, and evacuate. If unresponsive, care for as unresponsive victim (see chapter 11, "Neurologic Emergencies").

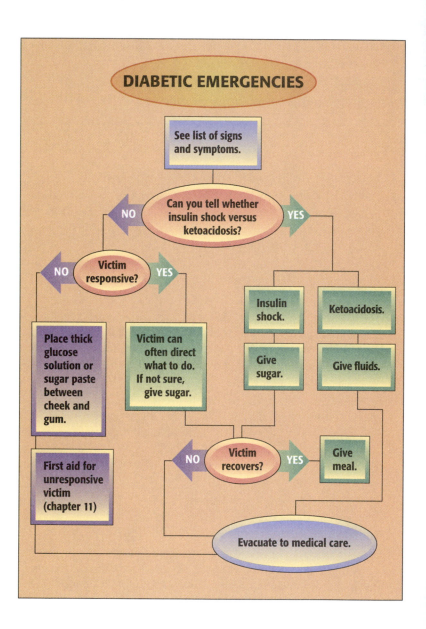

DIABETIC EMERGENCIES

See list of signs and symptoms.

Can you tell whether insulin shock versus ketoacidosis? — NO / YES

Victim responsive? — NO / YES

Place thick glucose solution or sugar paste between cheek and gum.

Victim can often direct what to do. If not sure, give sugar.

First aid for unresponsive victim (chapter 11)

Insulin shock.

Give sugar.

Ketoacidosis.

Give fluids.

Victim recovers? — NO / YES

Give meal.

Evacuate to medical care.

Allergic Reactions and Anaphylactic Shock

Allergic reactions may be mild and recurrent (e.g., hay fever, hives, and mild asthma) or sudden and severe (e.g., allergic swelling and severe asthmatic attacks). The most serious type is anaphylactic shock, an immediate and overwhelming allergic reaction seen in people who are extremely sensitive to insect stings, drugs, or foods.

Unlike milder allergic reactions such as hay fever, *anaphylactic shock* is a massive allergic reaction that overwhelms the body's systems with potentially fatal results. The majority of anaphylactic deaths result from inability to breathe because of swollen air passages. The next most common cause of death is from shock resulting from the collapse of the circulatory system. Wilderness first-aiders must attend to these crises as quickly as possible.

What to Look For

The victim suddenly (or, rarely, within hours) develops some or all of the following symptoms or signs while eating, after taking medicine, or after being stung by a bee or wasp:

➤ severe itching or hives

➤ sneezing, coughing, wheezing

➤ shortness of breath

➤ tightness and swelling of the throat

➤ tightness in the chest

➤ dramatic swelling of the face, tongue, and/or mouth

➤ vomiting, cramps, diarrhea

➤ convulsions, loss of responsiveness

What to Do

1. Act quickly. Every second counts.
2. Immediately perform the ABCs, with special attention to the airway.
3. *The only life-saving treatment is epinephrine!* It works by opening the airway, raising the blood pressure, and relieving swelling. If the victim or someone else in the party has a physician-prescribed epinephrine kit, administer it immediately according to the directions on the kit. Monitor the victim's condition every few minutes; if the victim's condition gets worse or there is no improvement after 3 minutes, give another injection of epinephrine.

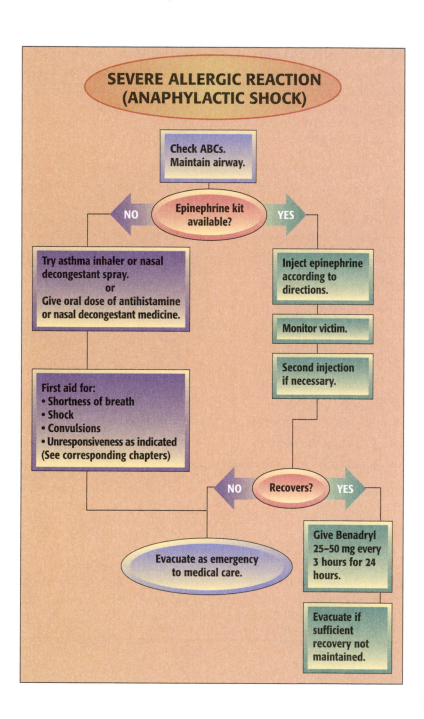

SEVERE ALLERGIC REACTION (ANAPHYLACTIC SHOCK)

Check ABCs. Maintain airway.

Epinephrine kit available?

NO

Try asthma inhaler or nasal decongestant spray.
or
Give oral dose of antihistamine or nasal decongestant medicine.

First aid for:
• Shortness of breath
• Shock
• Convulsions
• Unresponsiveness as indicated
(See corresponding chapters)

YES

Inject epinephrine according to directions.

Monitor victim.

Second injection if necessary.

Recovers?

NO

Evacuate as emergency to medical care.

YES

Give Benadryl 25–50 mg every 3 hours for 24 hours.

Evacuate if sufficient recovery not maintained.

4. If you don't have epinephrine,
   - use an asthma inhaler or nasal decongestant spray, or
   - give a dose of an antihistamine or nasal decongestant medication.

5. Give first aid for unresponsiveness (see pages 169–173) and/or seizures (see pages 179–180) as necessary.

6. Keep a conscious victim sitting up to help breathing; place an unconscious victim in the recovery position (see page 172).

7. After the victim improves, give 25–50 mg of Benadryl™ (1–2 of the over-the-counter capsules) every 3 hours for 24 hours (or longer if hives or other symptoms recur after stopping the Benadryl™).

8. If there is no improvement, evacuate rapidly.

MILD ALLERGIC REACTIONS

Allergic Rhinitis   Allergic rhinitis affects the nose, sinuses, and eyes. There are two main types: hay fever, due to windborne pollen and occurring only at certain seasons of the year; and perennial rhinitis, due to substances present year round, such as house dust, mites, feathers, animal dander, or molds.

What to Look For

➤ itching of the nose, roof of mouth, throat, and eyes

➤ stuffy, runny nose; runny eyes

➤ sneezing

What to Do

1. Avoid the cause, if known and if possible.

2. Give nonprescription or prescription oral antihistamines or antihistamine/decongestant combinations. The main drawbacks are drowsiness and a tendency to raise the blood pressure.

HIVES

Hives can result from allergy to a drug, insect sting or bite, or food (particularly eggs, nuts, fruit, or shellfish). They occasionally occur during a viral infection.

What to Look For

➤ pink, blotchy, itchy bumps on the skin (wheals) that range in size from less than ½ inch to several inches in diameter, and may be localized or cover the entire body

➤ occasional massive, itchy swelling of a lip, eyelid, hand, or foot

What to Do

1. Hives may precede anaphylactic shock (see above).

2. Most cases are self-limited and last only a few days to a week. Nonprescription antihistamines such as Benadryl are usually effective.

CHAPTER 14

Genitourinary Problems

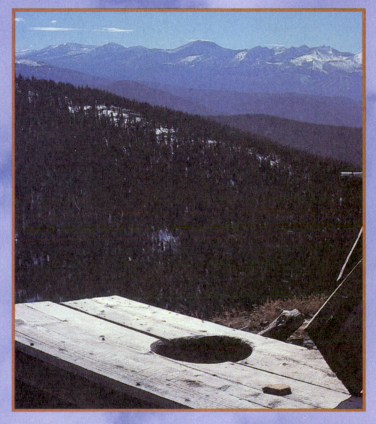

**Female Problems • Emergency Delivery • Pregnancy and
Wilderness Travel–General Considerations • Male Problems •
Guidelines for Evacuation of Genitourinary Problems**

Problems of the genitourinary tract can cause life-threatening bleeding, as with a tubal pregnancy; severe pain, as with a kidney stone; debilitating symptoms, as with a bladder infection; alarming symptoms, as with bloody urine or heavy uterine bleeding; serious illness, as with a kidney infection; or unexpected surprise, such as premature labor and delivery. As discussed in chapter 12, pain usually cannot be attributed to a specific cause, but with other symptoms, even the first-aider can arrive at a reasonable idea of the problem, which helps in the decision of when and how to get the victim to medical care. This section is meant to serve as a reference for these problems, not uncommon in the healthy, active group that travels in remote areas.

Female Problems
GENITAL PROBLEMS

Vaginitis   Vaginitis occurs when the normal balance of microbes in the vagina is altered, resulting in an irritating vaginal discharge. Common causes are infections by yeasts, bacteria, or protozoa (trichomonas). While uncomfortable, vaginal infections are not dangerous and do not require evacuation from the wilderness.

What to Look For

➤ vulvar soreness, burning or itching, redness

➤ increased vaginal discharge

➤ pain with urination

What to Do

1. Wear cotton underwear and loose-fitting pants.

2. Irrigate the vulva with clean water several times daily to remove the irritating discharge, then dry with a towel.

3. Use vaginal antifungal medication (nonprescription: clotrimazole [Gynelotrimin™] or miconazole [Monistat™]), which are highly effective against yeast vaginitis (the most common variety) and partially effective against trichomonas.

Vulvar Irritation–Allergic Vulvitis   Allergic vulvitis occurs when the vulva comes in contact with a substance that causes an allergic reaction, such as poison oak resin. Chemicals in clothing (detergents, fabric softeners, and scented sanitary napkins) can also irritate the vulva.

What to Look For

➤ vulvar soreness, burning, or itching *not* associated with increased vaginal discharge

➤ vulvar redness

➤ pain with urination

What to Do

1. Avoid further contact with the irritating substance.

2. Wash the vulva with clean water and mild soap; rinse generously.

3. Apply hydrocortisone cream (nonprescription) 3 times daily.

PROBLEMS WITH URINATION

Pain with urination, in the absence of vaginitis, vulvitis, and genital sores, is caused by a urinary tract infection.

What to Look For

➤ frequent, burning urination (strong urge with only small amounts of urine)

➤ low abdominal pain, cramping, and burning with urination

➤ cloudy or bloody urine

➤ foul-smelling urine

What to Do

1. Drink a lot of water.

2. Drink acidic fluids or juices.

3. Take vitamin C to acidify the urine.

4. Avoid sexual intercourse.

Most antibiotics become concentrated in the urine and will treat these infections. Begin a 3-day course. If pain while urinating is accompanied by fever, flank pain, pus or blood in the urine, nausea, or vomiting, seek medical help immediately.

VAGINAL BLEEDING AND MENSTRUAL IRREGULARITY

Missed Menses   Temporary absence of periods from lack of ovulation are common in menstruating women, especially in the teens and forties.

What to Look For

A history of unprotected intercourse, breast tenderness and nausea, or "morning sickness," may indicate pregnancy.

What to Do

1. If pregnancy is likely, see "Pregnancy and Wilderness Travel," later in this chapter.

2. A missed period usually requires no treatment. Consult a doctor if periods do not occur for 3 months.

Heavy or Prolonged Bleeding   Heavy or prolonged bleeding may occur after a missed period or in a woman with irregular periods.

What to Look For

➤ length of time since last period

➤ recent history of unprotected sex to suggest risk of pregnancy

➤ amount and duration of bleeding

➤ pale skin, nail, lips

➤ weakness

➤ signs and symptoms of shock (see page 150)

What to Do

1. Have the woman rest until bleeding decreases to a normal menstrual flow.

2. Give generous amounts of fluids to drink.

3. Seek medical attention if
   • bleeding saturates a pad every 3 hours or less for a 24-hour period.
   • the woman becomes pale and weak.

Bleeding on Hormonal Contraceptives   Irregular light bleeding is common on low-dose birth control pills. If no pills were missed, have the woman continue taking them daily as directed. If a pill was missed, give two the next day, and make sure the woman uses condoms or abstains from sex for the rest of the pill pack.

Erratic bleeding with Norplant™ and Depo-Provera™ is normal.

Bleeding with Pregnancy   Bleeding in pregnancy of less than 12 weeks' duration occurs with threatened miscarriage, miscarriage in progress, and ectopic pregnancy. Bleeding in a pregnancy of more than 12 weeks' duration occurs with miscarriage, labor, and abnormalities of the placenta.

What to Look For

➤ length of time since last period

➤ amount of bleeding

➤ low abdominal pain

➤ signs and symptoms of shock (see page 150)

What to Do

If a woman is less than 12 weeks pregnant, and bleeding remains light and painless, have her avoid physical exertion until the bleeding stops. She should abstain from sex until three weeks after the bleeding stops.

Seek medical attention or evacuate if

1. There is heavy bleeding.

2. Tissue (purple and spongy) passes vaginally.

3. There is low abdominal pain.

4. Pregnancy is longer than 12 weeks.

5. The victim becomes weak, pale, or her mental status is altered.

LOW ABDOMINAL PAIN

Low abdominal pain in women arises in the pelvic organs, intestines, or urinary tracts. A precise cause cannot be determined in the wilderness, so if the symptoms do not subside or if the woman is obviously sick and becoming worse, seek medical care.

Pain Due to Infections

What to Look For

➤ low abdominal pain

➤ fever

➤ nausea and vomiting

➤ diarrhea

What to Do

1. Intestinal infection: when pain coincides with fever, nausea, vomiting, and diarrhea, give as much fluid as tolerated. (See chapter 12, "Abdominal Emergencies.")

2. Pelvic infection: if the woman has increasing or constant pain, fever, nausea, and vomiting, seek medical attention. Maintain hydration with frequent sips of water.

Pain with Internal Bleeding from Ruptured Cyst or Ectopic Pregnancy

What to Look For

➤ low or generalized abdominal pain

➤ nausea

➤ signs of blood loss or shock (see page 150): pale color, weakness, dizziness on standing, rapid pulse, confusion

What to Do

1. Keep the woman lying at rest.

2. Have her walk out if capable and there is no possibility of timely help.

3. If she is unable to walk, send for help and evacuate.

Pain Associated with Pregnancy

What to Look For

➤ time since last period

➤ recurring pains

➤ signs of blood loss or shock

What to Do

1. Mild cramping in pregnancy without bleeding does not require treatment.

2. For pain with bleeding in pregnancy, follow the advice given for bleeding only (see above).

3. A woman more than 5 months pregnant who gets cramps lasting about 30 seconds every 15 minutes may be in labor. Have her drink a quart of water over 20 minutes—hydration tends to reduce preterm contractions. If the contractions do not subside over the next hour, evacuate to medical care.

Emergency Delivery

In case of delivery, have the woman lie or squat in a clean area. Place your hand firmly over the baby's head, applying gentle pressure to pre-

Emergency delivery

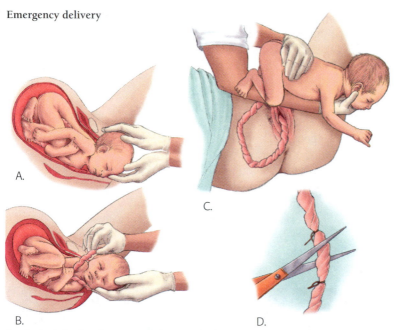

A.

C.

B.

D.

A. Control the head to control the speed of delivery and avoid large tears of the mother's peroneal area. If the head is still enveloped in the sac of amniotic fluid that is bulging out, nick or tear the sac to release the fluid.
B. If the cord is wrapped around the baby's neck, unloop it.
C. Hold the baby head down, rub dry to stimulate breathing. Pat on the back if necessary to stimulate cry. Wrap the baby in clothing to keep warm and place on mother's stomach.
D. Tie the cord in two locations. Cut between the ties. Wait for a lengthening of the cord and a small gush of blood that indicates placental separation, then pull gently on the cord. If the placenta does not come, wait a few minutes and try again. After the placenta is out, massage the lower abdomen firmly. The uterus can be felt as a hard ball through the abdominal wall.

vent it from being delivered too fast. When the infant is delivered, tie off the umbilical cord firmly with clean shoelaces or nylon cord in two places, and cut in between. Hold the baby upside down and tap or rub the back until the newborn breathes. Dry the baby and wrap to keep warm. The placenta normally comes out within 15 minutes after delivery. After a gush of ½–1 cup of blood, indicating separation of the placenta from the wall of the uterus, ask the woman to "push" (as if she were trying to go to the bathroom). If the placenta has not come out within 30 minutes, try massaging the lower abdomen. After the placenta comes out, grasp the abdomen over the uterus, at about the level of the umbilicus, and massage firmly and deeply for a minute or two, until the uterus feels like a firm ball. If vaginal bleeding becomes heavy, repeat the uterine massage.

Pregnancy and Wilderness Travel– General Considerations

A woman without major medical problems who exercises regularly before and during pregnancy, and who does not have a "high risk" pregnancy, can continue moderate exertion throughout pregnancy without risk to herself or her fetus.

Overheating in the first 12 weeks of pregnancy is associated with abnormal fetal development. In hot climates, pregnant women should maintain adequate hydration, pace themselves appropriately, and wear suitable clothing for their activities. They should avoid hot tubs.

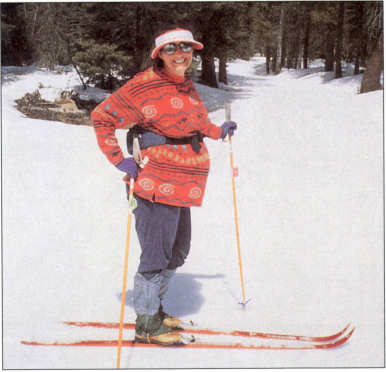

Exercise at moderate altitude is safe in pregnancy if there is no risk of trauma to the fetus.

Pregnant women should avoid any activity with a risk of abdominal trauma after the fourth month. Pregnant women may wish to stay below 16,000 feet due to a possible association of higher altitudes with birth defects. They should not travel to the wilderness within three weeks of the due date because of the risk of labor, and should refrain from scuba diving, as it is dangerous to the fetus.

Water treated with iodine is safe to drink for a few weeks during pregnancy. An alternative method using chlorine, filtration, or heat for disinfection must be used for a longer wilderness stay (see appendix C).

A pregnant woman planning international travel must get advice from her doctor about vaccinations and medications that are contraindicated in pregnancy.

Male Problems

Genitourinary problems in males are rarely life-threatening but are likely to be uncomfortable or worrisome enough that the victim will want to see a doctor.

PROBLEMS WITH URINATION

Painful Urination   Burning during urination usually indicates an infection.

What to Look For

➤ frequent, painful urination with only small amounts of urine, usually indicating an infection in the bladder

➤ yellow or white pus at the end of the penis, seen before urination in the morning or as stains on the underwear, indicates a sexually transmitted infection of the urethra

What to Do

1. For bladder/urinary tract infection, see below.

2. For sexually transmitted urethritis, have the man avoid sex and seek medical care.

Bloody Urine   This is frightening, but is not generally an emergency.

What to Look For

➤ pink or red urine

➤ severe back or flank pain, suggesting a kidney stone or infection

➤ fever, suggesting an infection in the prostate or kidneys

➤ inability to urinate, possibly resulting from a blood clot in the bladder

What to Do

1. Give several extra quarts of water per day unless the victim is unable to urinate.
2. Have the victim walk out if no pain or fever.

Frequent Urination   This may be a symptom of infection, urinary obstruction, or diabetes with elevated blood sugar.

What to Look For

➤ fever, chills, and back pain with burning on urination, indicating an infection

➤ constant thirst, drinking and urinating large volumes, suggesting diabetes

➤ frequent small amounts of urine with a sense that the bladder cannot be emptied completely and fullness in lower abdomen, suggesting infection or urinary obstruction

What to Do

1. Increase intake of water and fruit juices unless there is possible obstruction.
2. Give vitamin C (500 mg 3 times daily), which makes the urine acid and slows bacterial growth.
3. If infection is likely and the person has an antibiotic, he should take it.
4. Seek medical care (see "Guidelines for Evacuation of Genitourinary Problems" at the end of this chapter).

Inability to Urinate   Obstruction occurs in older men with enlarged prostates, and is often induced by prolonged sitting during travel or by medications such as antihistamines and cold remedies. It may occur in young men with prior surgery on the urinary tract or after pelvic injury.

What to Look For

➤ painfully full bladder

➤ inability to pass any urine or frequent dribbling of small amounts of urine without relief

What to Do

1. Stop any medications for allergies, congestion/colds, stomach cramps, motion sickness; stop over-the-counter sleep medication.
2. Limit fluid intake.
3. Take the man for a walk.
4. Listen to running water, place the man's hand in pot of warm water, or have him sit in warm water.
5. If he is still unable to urinate, evacuate.

GENITAL PROBLEMS

Testicular Pain   Sudden onset of pain and swelling in the testicle of a young man (less than 25 years old) means it is twisted (torsion) and requires surgery within 24 hours to prevent damage to the testicle. Gradual onset of pain and swelling in an adult more likely indicates infection (epididymitis) than torsion.

What to Look For

➤ severe pain in testicle, often spreading to groin or lower abdomen on the same side: may cause vomiting

➤ testicle is firm and swollen

➤ urine can pass but may be hard to start due to pain.

TWISTED TESTICLE	ADVANCED PROCEDURE

What to Do

The testicle can sometimes be untwisted by hand. Try rotating the testicle 180°, first in one direction then the other, while exerting gentle traction in a vertical axis with the man standing. If relief is obtained, it will be rapid.

Pain and Swelling of Foreskin   In uncircumcised men or boys, the foreskin may become inflamed and cannot be pulled over the end of the penis.

What to Look For

➤ redness, swelling, and pain of the foreskin; inability to retract or extend the foreskin freely

➤ pus or whitish mucus under the foreskin

What to Do

1. Have the man gently compress the swollen tissue and try to move the foreskin.

2. Have him wash the area daily with mild soap, cleaning beneath the foreskin as well.

3. Have him dry the area, then apply an antifungal cream and/or antibiotic ointment.

4. Administer an antibiotic, if possible.

5. If the man is unable to urinate or to relieve the pain and swelling, seek medical help.

KIDNEY STONE

A kidney stone is one of the most common causes of *sudden* severe flank and abdominal pain.

What to Look For

➤ sudden onset of pain in flank on one side, often spreading to lower abdomen, groin, or testicle

➤ severe pain causing restlessness and vomiting

➤ bloody urine

What to Do

1. Administer pain medication.

2. Increase fluid intake.

3. Evacuate if severe pain or fever.

Guidelines for Evacuation of Genitourinary Problems

Evacuate for

- urinary obstruction with inability to urinate
- urinary symptoms with fever, chills, and back pain
- sudden testicular pain
- swelling, redness, and pain around shaft of penis or scrotum

  No evacuation is necessary (the victim may walk out) for

- bloody urine
- frequent urination without fever
- pus discharge from or sores on penis

CHAPTER 15

Physical and Environmental Hazards

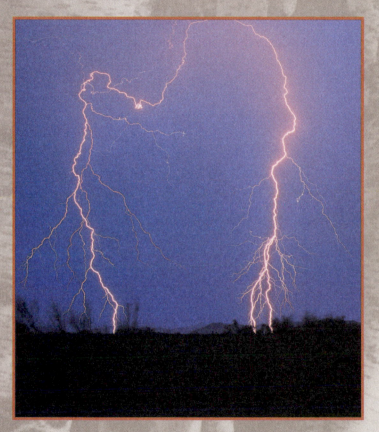

Acute Mountain Sickness (AMS) • **Cold Injury** •

Heat Exposure • **Lightning Injury**

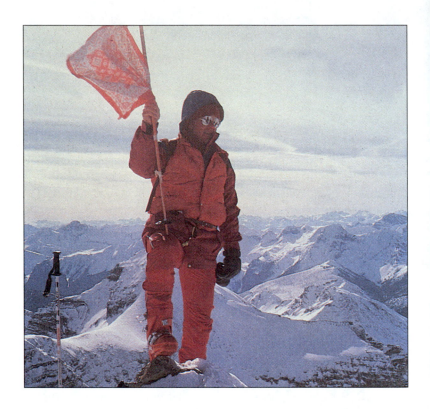

The environment and its effects on the body distinguish wilderness from urban first aid. Altitude, cold, heat, wind, rain, lightning, soaking wetness, and parching dryness not only cause injuries and illnesses but incidentally affect those that occur in the wilderness. An injury that might have little significance in the city becomes important if it stops a person from hiking and exposes him or her to a cold night out. Both the severity of the elements and the length of time for which the injured person is exposed may affect the outcome: A night spent with a broken ankle when the temperature is 60°F, with neither rain nor wind, may be uncomfortable and painful but will be survived. The same broken ankle incurred in winter at 12,000 feet on the windy slopes of a mountain, far from camp and with no way to call for help, could be fatal.

It is, therefore, important to understand not only the management of individual injuries but the effects of the surrounding environment on an injured person. How will the temperature, altitude, and weather affect the outcome? And what must be done to prevent further injury by protecting the person from the heat or cold, the wind or rain? What must you do to provide food and fluids to maintain the victim's strength? How can you improvise a shelter? The answers may mean the difference between life and death. But first you must understand how the environment affects the body.

ACCLIMATIZATION

Acclimatization comprises the physiological changes in the body that compensate for hypoxia at altitudes above 8,000 feet (2,500 meters) and allow humans to live, work, and exercise with what little oxygen is available. It proceeds at different rates in different people. Acclimatization is best achieved through slow, progressive ascent with rest or descent if symptoms persist.

IMMEDIATE CHANGES OF ACCLIMATIZATION

The rate and depth of breathing increase to improve oxygen delivery to the blood; the heart beats more quickly and strongly, increasing the flow of blood and transport of oxygen.

LATE CHANGES OF ACCLIMATIZATION

The bone marrow produces more red cells to carry oxygen; an increase in the number of capillaries improves oxygen supply to muscles and other tissues.

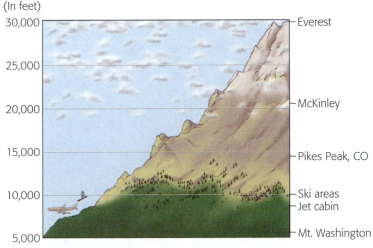

(In feet)

- 30,000 — Everest
- 25,000
- 20,000 — McKinley
- 15,000 — Pikes Peak, CO
- 10,000 — Ski areas / Jet cabin
- 5,000 — Mt. Washington

Various altitudes

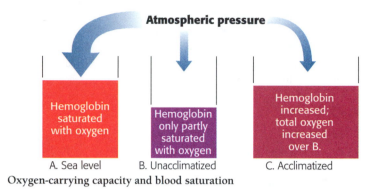

Oxygen-carrying capacity and blood saturation

TYPES OF ALTITUDE SICKNESS

1. Mild to moderate
   - Acute mountain sickness (AMS): Symptoms develop within 6 to 48 hours after ascent to altitudes above 8,000 feet; usually improves in 36 to 72 hours if there is no further ascent.
2. Severe
   - *High altitude pulmonary edema* (HAPE): Fluid collects in the lungs.
   - *High altitude cerebral edema* (HACE): The brain swells due to accumulation of fluid.

Acute Mountain Sickness (AMS)

Acute mountain sickness is caused by diminished oxygen pressure in the air at altitudes above 8,000 feet, due to diminished oxygen in the blood (hypoxia). It strikes those who ascend too high too fast and those who have not acclimatized to high altitude. AMS is usually cured by descent to a lower altitude.

PREDICTING AMS

No one can predict who will suffer from AMS, how severe it will be, or when it will occur. Those who have suffered AMS before are more likely to suffer again, and at a similar altitude. Fitness and training guarantee no protection, both sexes succumb equally, and no age is exempt. The young appear more prone, regardless of fitness and rate of ascent.

PREVENTION

Climbers should allow ample time to acclimatize at various levels of ascent. AMS is more likely to occur the higher, the faster, the harder, and the longer the climb. Cold and wind, fear, fatigue, dehydration, strenuous exercise soon after ascent, and upper respiratory infections all predispose to AMS.

HIGH ALTITUDE CLIMBING

Mild symptoms of AMS may develop at 6,000 feet, but are more likely above 8,000 feet. Above 13,000 feet climbers and trekkers on multi-day trips should gain sleeping altitude at about 1,000 feet per day. The motto is: "Climb high, sleep low."

Climbers who become sick and do not improve with rest must descend 1,000–3,000 feet as quickly as possible. Be aware of climbers who acclimatize poorly. They may be headed for trouble.

Drink 4–5 quarts of fluid daily, enough to produce clear, copious urine. Dark (concentrated) urine usually indicates an inadequate fluid intake.

Alcohol, sedatives, and sleeping pills depress respiratory ventilation at night and increase the likelihood of disturbed sleep. Eat a high-calorie, high-carbohydrate diet.

MILD AMS

Mild AMS has vague, ill-defined symptoms but can drift subtly into severe altitude sickness, which can kill. Symptoms and signs of mild AMS occur within 6 to 48 hours of arrival at altitude.

What to Look For

➤ a generalized headache that often develops during the night and is present on waking; by day, the victim may feel light-headed

➤ unusual tiredness out of proportion to the activity

➤ appetite loss and nausea

➤ restless sleep with irregular breathing

➤ shortness of breath with exertion

➤ the face is swollen, with bags under the eyes; rings on fingers feel tight

TABLE 15.1

Characteristics of Altitude Illnesses

	AMS	HAPE	HACE
Elevation	Above 6,000 ft.	Usually above 10,000 ft.	Above 12,000 ft.
Time after ascent	1–2 days	3–4 days, possibly later	4–7 days, possibly later
Symptoms	Result from hypoxia and include headache, sleep disturbance, fatigue, shortness of breath, dizziness, loss of appetite, vomiting	Caused by pulmonary fluid and include shortness of breath, dry cough, mild chest pain, weakness, insomnia, rapid pulse, cyanosis, rales (crackles) or gurgling sounds	Caused by swelling of the brain and include severe headache (unrelieved), vomiting, Cheynes-Strokes breathing (irregular breathing pattern followed by breathing stops), staggering gait, inability to balance, unconsciousness
First aid	• Stop ascending or go down. • Drink fluids. • Rest. • Take aspirin or ibuprofen. • Responds to Diamox™.	• Descend at least 2,000 ft. • Seek medical attention *immediately.*	• Descend as soon as possible; 1,000 ft. minimum, 3,000 ft. if possible or until symptoms disappear. • Seek medical attention *immediately.*

Notes: AMS = acute mountain sickness; HAPE = high-altitude pulmonary edema; HACE = high-altitude cerebral edema.
HAPE and HACE occur when reduced oxygen causes capillary leakage and body-tissue swelling. Both conditions are life-threatening.

What to Do

1. Rest and **do not go any higher.**

2. Wait and see. If headache or shortness of breath increase despite taking aspirin or acetaminophen and resting, diagnose severe AMS and descend 1,000 to 3,000 feet, or until the victim feels better.

3. Give acetazolamide (brand name Diamox™), for the prevention and treatment of mild AMS symptoms.

4. Give dexamethasone (brand name Decadron™) for severe headache. Travelers who have already experienced altitude symptoms should consider prescriptions for these medications before going to altitude again.

Mild AMS may turn slowly into severe altitude sickness. Life-threatening symptoms can develop within hours, and frequently do so at night, when descending is more difficult. It is better to misdiagnose the condition too early as severe AMS and descend than to underestimate mild AMS.

SEVERE ALTITUDE SICKNESS

High Altitude Pulmonary Edema (HAPE)   In HAPE the lungs become waterlogged, hindering the passage of oxygen into the blood. Victims can drown in their own fluid. HAPE usually starts above 10,000 feet but can occur at lower altitudes; it begins 36 to 72 hours after arriving at altitude and is cured by descent.

What to Look For

➤ shortness of breath, which occurs with slight exertion and is even present at rest. The victim needs to sit up to breathe comfortably.

➤ cough, at first dry, then producing frothy, pink (blood-stained) sputum

➤ rattly or crackling and moist breathing and coughing

➤ cyanosis, when lips, face, and fingernails look blue at rest (compare victim's color to a fit companion or yourself in natural light, not in a tent)

➤ rapid pulse, more than 100 beats per minute at rest

What to Do

1. Descend; this is the most important principle of treatment.

2. Give oxygen if available.

3. Commence treatment in a portable compression chamber.

4. Administer acetazolamide and/or nifedipine in accordance with prearranged instructions.

High Altitude Cerebral Edema (HACE)   HACE usually occurs above 12,000 feet. It may accompany HAPE and can kill quickly. Symptoms of HACE and HAPE may overlap.

What to Look For

➤ severe, constant, throbbing headache, like a bad toothache or migraine; no relief from acetaminophen, codeine, or a night's rest

➤ incoordination (ataxia); the victim staggers as if drunk and fumbles fine movements and cannot walk a straight line with the heel of one foot against the toes of the other. If ataxia is severe, the victim cannot sit upright without support.

➤ extreme fatigue, not reversed by rest. The person won't talk, eat, or drink and is apathetic and isolated, irritable, and confused. The person may hallucinate, hear voices, or see nonexistent companions.

Note: Ataxia and fatigue occur in other conditions such as hypothermia (check the temperature), alcohol intoxication (smell the breath), and opiate drug abuse (look for pinpoint pupils).

➤ vomiting, which, combined with the inability to drink, may lead to severe dehydration. Urine becomes scanty and dark yellow.

➤ coma, where the person becomes unarousable and unresponsive, drifts into unconsciousness and may die

What to Do

1. Descend. This usually cures severe altitude sickness rapidly. Do not delay descent because of night, inconvenience, trying drugs or oxygen, or in expectation of a mountain rescue team or helicopter—unless descending through difficult terrain in the dark will cause unwarranted danger to the whole party. The victim, always accompanied and perhaps carried, should descend at least 1,000 to 3,000 feet. Even a modest descent can save a life. The greater and faster the descent, the swifter the recovery. Once down, the person should stay down.

2. Treat for several hours in a Gamow bag. This may be life-saving under extreme circumstances and may buy time while a rescue operation is being mounted. (Climbing parties going to extreme altitudes should consider being equipped with a bag.)

3. Have the victim sit propped up to improve breathing. Keep the person warm and relaxed. Cold and anxiety aggravate AMS.

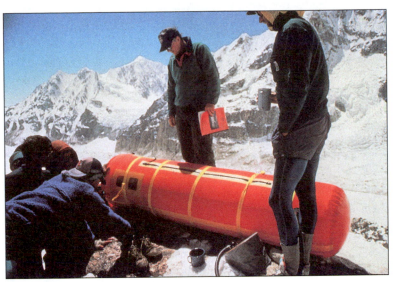

Gamow bag

4. Drink at least 4 to 5 quarts or liters of fluid daily, enough to maintain a copious flow of clear urine.

5. Acetazolamide and dexamethasone in small doses reduce significantly the chance of getting AMS and its severity should it occur. But do not rely on drugs to allow a rapid ascent; this is dangerous.

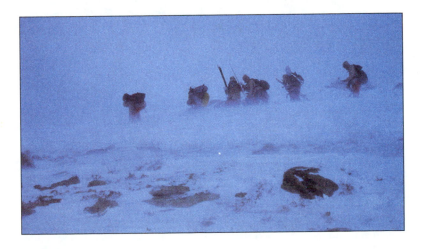

Cold Injury
HYPOTHERMIA

Hypothermia is general cooling of the body core when more heat is lost than is produced. *Frostbite* is local freezing of the skin and flesh. *Immersion injury* occurs in water in the absence of freezing. Both hypothermia and frostbite may coexist, but treat hypothermia first because it can kill. Hypothermia is exacerbated by inadequate clothing and exhaustion. Anxiety, injury, drugs, poor nutrition, and alcohol consumption predispose to its development.

Wetness and wind are a lethal combination that chill a person more rapidly than dry cold. Heat loss is 25 times more rapid in water than in dry, still air. Wetness does not come only from falling into a lake—sweat-soaked clothes are as potent a cause of heat loss. The conditions for hypothermia, therefore, exist in all seasons of the year. The hiker exposed to a sudden summer hailstorm while wearing only a T-shirt and cutoff jeans is more likely to become hypothermic than a well-dressed cross-country skier in the winter. Substituting dry clothes for wet may be the most important first step in the first aid of all cold victims.

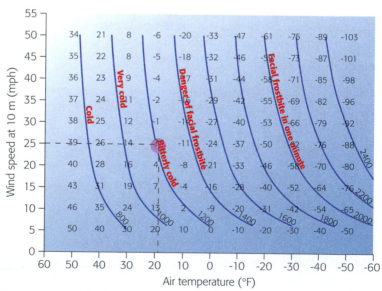

The point at which a horizontal line from the wind speed scale meets a vertical line from the air temperature scale indicates the equivalent temperature. With a wind speed of 25 mph and an air temperature of 20° F, the equivalent temperature is 0° F.

The windchill factor (see chart on page 230) shows the cooling effects of wind at any given temperature and wind speed. It is, however, important to realize that windchill affects only the exposed parts of the body, usually the face and neck. Wearing windproof clothing and covering the face with a mask and goggles can reduce or eliminate the effects of windchill, except under the most severe circumstances.

P R E V E N T I O N

Plan carefully, even for the shortest outdoor expedition, and carry a water/wind-repellent shell, pile jacket, hat and mittens, matches, and a space blanket or tarp for shelter. If the weather changes, be prepared to abandon the original plan and take an easier, shorter route home, or bivouac.

Watch for early signs of hypothermia, and act promptly to avert it. Gauge the day's activity to the party's weakest member. Being exhausted, hungry, dehydrated, or demoralized prevents a proper response to cold and hastens the onset of hypothermia. Even after exertion stops, body temperature may plummet because heat loss continues while heat production decreases sharply. Evaporation of sweat is the most important source of heat loss during exercise. Avoidance of sweating, therefore, with appropriately ventilated clothing is important to maintain comfort and avoid excessive heat loss.

Children and adolescents lose heat faster than adults because their surface area is large in proportion to their weight, and generally they have less subcutaneous fat.

Means of Heat Loss

- Convection: heat is carried away from the body by currents of air or water
- Conduction: direct transfer of heat from the body to a colder object (e.g., wet clothes or cold ground)
- Evaporation of sweat or water from the surface of the skin
- Radiation: the loss of heat from a warm body to a surrounding colder environment. This is independent of wind or contact. Radiative heat loss is significant in cold, dark, cloudless nights.

Sources of Heat Gain

- Radiation: heat from the sun or a fire
- Exercise: 75% of muscular energy is produced as heat; exercise, therefore, rewarms the body.

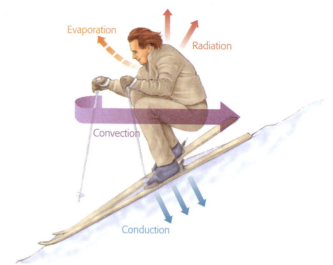

Sources of heat loss

- Shivering: shivering can increase body metabolism fivefold but consumes energy and oxygen in achieving this.

- Food: provides calories for basic body functions and exercise. Carbohydrates provide energy quickly; protein provides greater energy, but more slowly and at the expense of more body energy.

- Blood vessel constriction: skin blood vessels constrict, thereby keeping warm blood circulating in the core, where it is most needed by the vital organs (brain, heart, liver, kidneys) and reducing heat loss through the skin.

- Insulation: prevents heat loss but does not by itself produce heat. Water, an excellent heat conductor, reduces the insulating value of most fabrics. Wool, polypropylene, and pile insulate well by trapping air in the interstices of the fibers, which do not collapse when wet. The more layers of clothing the better the insulation. Windproof, water-repellent fabrics, as an outer layer of clothing, trap warm air in the inner layers and diminish heat loss by convection, conduction, and evaporation.

MILD HYPOTHERMIA

The core temperature of the body will range from 35°C to 33°C (95°F to 91°F).

What to Look For

➤ shivering, the first sign of body cooling. Shivering later becomes uncontrollable.

➤ uncharacteristic behavior: the person can still talk, but grumbles and mumbles about feeling cold. Such behavior may be obvious only to someone who knows the victim. Inappropriate excitement or lethargy, poor judgment, and poor decision making are common. The person becomes confused and may hallucinate.

➤ stiff muscles and cramps; these cause uncoordinated movements, so the victim fumbles and stumbles and may not be able to walk along a straight line for 50 to 100 feet.

➤ cold, pale and blue-gray skin owing to constricted blood vessels

What to Do

1. Find shelter out of the wind.

2. Light a fire or stove, change the victim's wet clothes, add layers to increase insulation, give some food and a hot drink.

3. If the victim is shivering strongly, remove wet clothing and allow shivering to continue inside a sleeping bag, keeping the victim well insulated from the ground. *Note:* Putting a rescuer in a sleeping bag with the victim is not always the best thing to do. Warming the skin stops shivering, the most effective internal method of rewarming. Get the victim out of wet clothes. Provide maximum insulation and shelter, and allow shivering to do the rewarming. It may be better to have one person in two sleeping bags than two people in one bag.

4. Give warm, sweet liquids.

5. Do not delay. If the victim responds to rest and warmth, he or she may be able to descend to a camp or hut to be thoroughly warmed.

6. Never leave a hypothermic victim alone.

SEVERE HYPOTHERMIA

With severe hypothermia, the body's core temperature falls below 32°C (90°F).

Because few people carry a low-reading thermometer in the wilderness, a more practical way of differentiating between mild and severe hypothermia is to classify victims as shivering and nonshivering. A victim who is conscious and shivering is "mildly" hypothermic. A barely

TABLE 15.2

Field Management
of Hypothermia

Assessment	Victim: Severity of hypothermia Group: Number, condition, strength, available equipment Circumstances: Weather, time of day, distance from help, etc.
Plan	Rewarming Shelter Communications/logistics Evacuation
Action	Shelter; clothing; food; heat sources; contacting help; preparation for stay or evacuation Treatment of associated injuries or illnesses

conscious victim who is so cold that he or she is no longer shivering is "severely" hypothermic.

What to Look For

➤ no shivering

➤ behavior changing from erratic to apathetic to unresponsive

➤ stiff muscles and uncoordinated movement

➤ weak, slow, irregular pulse

➤ slow breathing

➤ coma, with dilated pupils (It may be difficult to determine if the victim is alive or dead.)

What to Do (in the Field)

There are no effective methods for rewarming in the field; concentrate your efforts on reducing further heat loss.

1. The leader or most competent person in the group must take charge. Do not endanger other members of the party.

2. Shelter everyone, as well as the victim, from wind, rain, and snow and out of danger from avalanche or rock fall. Erect a tent, dig a snow hole, or build a lean-to.

3. Stop further heat loss. Remove wet or freezing clothing and dress the victim in dry clothes. Put the person in a sleeping bag, bivouac

sack, or a strong polyethylene bag and insulate him or her well from the cold ground.

4. Provide heat urgently to the victim's trunk during the first half-hour after rescue by whatever means are available—body-to-body contact, hot water bottles, chemical heating pads, hot rocks wrapped in clothing. Place the heat sources in the groin and armpits and alongside the neck. Always have clothing between a heat source and the skin.

5. Cover the victim's head with a wool cap to reduce heat loss.

What to Do (Rescue)

1. Leave at least one person to look after the victim. Send the strongest, most competent members of the party for help. Provide the location and the condition of the victim in a written message.

2. Having decided to stay put and await rescue, do not change your plan even if the victim improves. If you are forced to carry the person, insulate him or her well because cooling may continue during transportation.

3. If you must descend, choose the safest route that avoids ridges and windy places. If the victim is on an improvised stretcher or sled, handle gently; rough handling can induce ventricular fibrillation. Carry the victim with the head downhill to maintain blood pressure.

What to Do (Base Camp)

1. If rescue is impossible, or days away, use all available means to rewarm the victim slowly in a sleeping bag.

2. If the victim has become hypothermic over hours or days due to exposure, do not try rapid rewarming in a bath or in front of a fire.

3. Give the person plenty of warm, sweet liquids when he or she is able to drink. Hypothermic victims are often dehydrated and energy-depleted. You cannot expect to provide enough heat in warm drinks to rewarm a hypothermic person, but the hydration and usable energy are valuable, and the warmth will help build morale in the victim.

4. Be careful not to place warm objects (hot water bottles, chemical heating pads, etc.) directly on the victim's skin. Hypothermic skin burns at low temperatures.

DEEP HYPOTHERMIA

With deep hypothermia, the body's core temperature falls below 28°C (82°F).

The victim may appear dead, but declare a victim of hypothermia dead only after warming has been attempted. The person's pupils may be dilated and fixed, the limbs stiff, and the skin icy. Profoundly hypothermic persons cannot generate enough metabolic heat to rewarm themselves, despite good shelter and insulation. They cannot be rewarmed in the field but, once rescued, all hypothermic victims in whom there appears even a remote chance of recovery should be resuscitated. Protect and insulate them during transportation to prevent further heat loss. The only sure sign of death is failure to revive with rewarming. Victims have survived after several hours of rescue breathing and CPR.

IMMERSION HYPOTHERMIA

Immersion hypothermia differs from exposure hypothermia in its rapid onset and even faster rate of cooling. Heat is lost 25 times faster in water than in air because water is an excellent conductor of heat. The victim may drown in addition to becoming hypothermic.

Most people can swim less than 0.6 mile (1 km) in water at 50°F (10°C). Energetic swimming increases heat loss, while floating in a fetal position minimizes it. A personal flotation device (PFD) prolongs survival time threefold. Clothes decrease heat loss; wool insulates better than other materials when wet, and covering the head reduces heat loss by half.

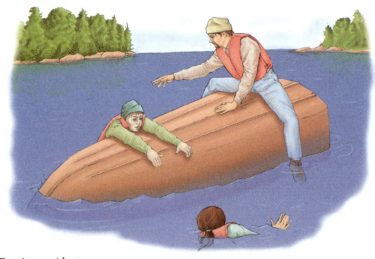

Boating accident scene

It is safer to stay with an overturned boat than to strike out for shore. A person will stay warmer out of the water, clinging to an over-turned boat—despite wind and rain—than staying immersed. Staying with the boat increases the chance of rescue. Unfortunately, despair is the overwhelming emotion among shipwreck victims, who are inclined not to bother with details of survival skills that can tip the balance from death to life.

In water colder than 45°F hypothermia can develop in less than an hour, but the more clothes the victim is wearing the slower the onset of hypothermia. Many victims drown because of a combination of cold, which reduces their ability to swim or float, and submersion. People who die within a few minutes of entering cold water do not die from hypothermia but from submersion, from waves splashing over the face, or from rapid changes in blood acidity induced by hyperventilation.

CPR must be started as soon as possible after the victim is removed from the water. (For criteria for starting and stopping CPR see pages 292–294.) If the victim is very cold it may not be possible to restart the heart until the person has been rewarmed in a hospital; but rescue efforts should continue until this has been done or there is clearly no hope of recovery.

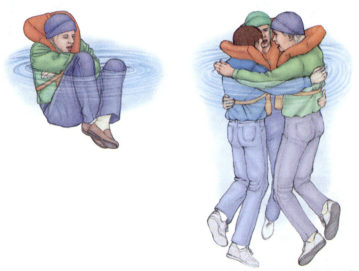

HELP or Huddle. A person wearing a flotation device can minimize heat loss and increase chances of survival by assuming the Heat Escape Lessening Posi-tion, or HELP (left), in which the knees are pulled up to the chest and the arms crossed. Groups of three or more can conserve heat by wrapping their arms around one another and pulling into a tight circle (right).

FROSTBITE

Frostbite is localized freezing of tissues, most commonly the face, hands, and feet. In severe cold weather the extremities are less likely to freeze if the core remains warm. Once frostbitten, the area may forever remain more susceptible to cold injury.

Factors that contribute to frostbite include wetness, contact with metal, prolonged exposure, dehydration, poor nutrition, extremely cold temperatures, and immobilization, whether by injury or circumstances. In severe cold, or if there is contact with metal, frostbite can occur in a minute. At high altitude the risk of frostbite is greater because there is less oxygen to nourish the tissues.

Types of Frostbite   *Frostnip* is a superficial injury involving the surface of the skin. It is easily treated by immediate warming, and there is no residual damage. *Superficial frostbite* involves all the layers of the skin but not the underlying fat, muscles, etc. It is associated with swelling and blisters filled with clear fluid. *Deep frostbite* involves the skin and underlying tissues to a variable depth, depending on the severity of the injury. The affected part has no feeling; blisters do not extend to the

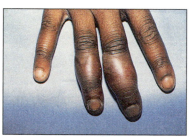

Frostbitten fingers, 6 hours after re-warming in 108°F water

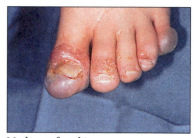

Moderate frostbite

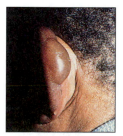

Frostbitten ear 8 hours old

tips of the digits and are blood filled; and the tissues remain cold even after attempts to rewarm.

What to Look For

➤ white, waxy skin that has no feeling and is wooden to the touch

➤ possible thawing, in which case
- the skin is soft and the part may appear gray or purple
- the skin tingles painfully
- blisters develop within a few hours

What to Do

1. Avoid a freeze-thaw-refreeze cycle. It is possible to walk with a frozen foot, but preferable not to walk with a foot that has thawed. If the hand is frozen and can be protected and kept warm, and the victim can walk out, thawing may not be harmful and may be un-avoidable. In many mountaineering accidents some thawing has occurred before the victim is first seen.

2. If you are more than 8 hours from help, allow the part to thaw. If the victim's boots are removed to allow thawing, it may be impossible to get them back on again because of the swelling.

3. Keep the part clean.

4. Cover the part with a dry, protective dressing.

5. Elevate the limb above the level of the heart to reduce swelling.

6. If thawing is inevitable, or if the victim is in a place from which transportation is assured, warm the frozen part in water at 102°F to 104°F for 30 to 40 minutes. Dry the part carefully and protect it from further damage.

7. Evacuate as soon as possible.

 DO NOT
- **rub with snow.**
- **break blisters.**
- **allow to refreeze.**
- **warm the part in front of a fire or heater. A burn may add to the damage. Rewarming can be very painful.**

P
R
E
V
E
N
T
I
O
N

To avoid frostbite,

- wear windproof, water-repellent clothing
- avoid wetness or handling metal with bare hands
- avoid tight clothes, boots, and crampons
- wear gaiters to keep snow out of boots
- pull a plastic bag over the foot next to the skin to act as a vapor barrier
- change socks frequently to keep feet dry
- carry spare dry socks that double as mittens
- warm feet or hands as soon as they begin to feel cold or lose feeling
- wear mittens rather than gloves, with a silk or polypropylene liner
- watch each other's faces for white patches of frostnip
- jump up and down, wiggle toes, flex ankles, clap hands, and swing arms if the feet or hands are becoming cold. Place a cold foot against the trunk of a warm, sympathetic companion

IMMERSION (TRENCH) FOOT

Immersion foot is a nonfreezing cold injury caused by prolonged exposure (average 3 days) to cold and wet, but without freezing. Mild numbness may progress to swelling, loss of feeling, and burning pain. Blisters develop in severe cases. The injury may occur in people rafting or kayaking in very cold water, or in sailors stranded for days in a life raft and unable to keep their feet out of water.

Prevent injury by keeping feet warm and dry, with frequent sock changes and foot hygiene. Rubber boots do not necessarily protect the feet since cold sweat may have the same effect as water.

Treat by elevating the feet and exposing them to the air. The burning feeling is relieved by cool air. Give analgesics as necessary.

In very severe cases, walking may be impossible due to pain, and evacuation is mandatory.

CHILBLAINS

Chilblains result from repeated exposure of bare skin to wet, wind, and cold; they cause red, itchy, tender, swollen skin, usually on the fingers. Chilblains are not a severe problem and can be prevented by wearing gloves.

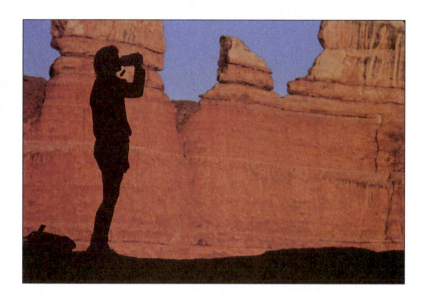

Heat Exposure

The body balances heat loss against heat gain to keep the core body temperature within narrow limits. Evaporation of sweat is the most important means of dissipating heat when exercising, but fluid and salt are also lost. With strenuous exercise in hot climates heat gain can exceed loss. Core temperature may rise, sometimes to dangerous levels.

Dehydration, factors that limit ability to sweat (certain skin diseases, extensive prior burns, some medications) or prior cardiovascular problems can predispose to heat illness. The same factors that affect heat loss apply to heat balance for heat illness.

Acclimatization to heat produces physiologic changes in the body over 3 to 10 days that allow greater comfort and ability to exercise or work in the heat. Acclimatization is stimulated by 1 to 1.5 hours of exercise a day in the heat.

P R E V E N T I O N
To avoid heat illness, anyone who is active in hot weather should drink when exercising, before feeling thirsty and after feeling satisfied. The person should drink water or a sports electrolyte solution every hour, enough to produce clear urine regularly during the day. For exercise lasting 2 to 3 hours, salt and glucose can be replaced after the exertion. For sustained exertion in the heat, glucose and salt must be replaced during exercise; this is best done by eating in addition to drinking (see appendix D). Salt food liberally or include salty snacks.

- Avoid heavy exercise in high temperatures and high humidity.
- Wear light-colored clothes that fit loosely and cover all sun-exposed skin surface.
- Avoid alcohol and caffeine; both increase loss of fluid.
- Be aware of the early symptoms—headache, nausea, muscle cramps.

HEAT EXHAUSTION

Heat exhaustion develops over hours or days due to water and electrolyte loss from sweating. It may also cause collapse or gradual exhaustion with an inability to continue exercise. The symptoms are nonspecific and often referred to as "summer flu" because of the resemblance to viral illness: headache, dizziness, fatigue, nausea, and vomiting.

What to Look For

➤ inability to continue exercise or work due to symptoms

➤ headache, nausea, dizziness, and weakness

➤ rapid pulse

➤ thirst and profuse sweating

➤ gooseflesh, chills, and pale skin

➤ normal or moderately raised temperature, 39°C (102°F) to 41°C (105°F); falls quickly with measures below

➤ low blood pressure; victim may faint

What to Do

1. Have the victim rest in the shade and maximize air circulation.
2. Have the victim remove excess clothing.

3. Wet the victim with cold water to increase evaporation.

4. Have the victim drink fluids .

5. For more severe cases add ¼ teaspoon salt and 6 teaspoons sugar to 1 liter of water (see appendix C).

HEATSTROKE

One type of heatstroke occurs in otherwise healthy, fit people of any age who undertake heavy exertion in hot climates (e.g., military training and warfare, endurance races and sporting events, and strenuous occupations).

A second type of heatstroke may also occur without exercise after several days of exposure to a heat wave. This usually occurs in people with chronic medical or psychiatric illness. Heatstroke results in sudden collapse with extreme elevation of body temperature, decreased mental status, and circulatory shock. It is a medical emergency that can kill.

What to Look For

➤ headache

➤ drowsiness, irritability, unsteadiness in victim; then sudden confusion, delirium, with convulsions and coma

➤ rapid pulse and low blood pressure

➤ dry or sweat-moistened hot skin

➤ temperature (preferably taken rectally) above 41°C (106°F) (do not attempt to take an oral temperature in a confused or combative person)

What to Do

1. Remove the victim from heat.

2. Remove all victim's clothing down to the underwear to accelerate cooling.

3. Effect immediate, rapid cooling by one of these methods:
   • Increase evaporation by sprinkling or spraying water on the skin (but is ineffective in high humidity); fan vigorously.
   • Immerse the victim's body in a stream or a cold bath.
   • Place cold packs on the neck, abdomen, armpits, and groin.

4. Stop cooling when the rectal temperature falls to 39°C (102°F) or when mental status improves.

5. Monitor the victim's temperature frequently, because it may rise again.

Note: Heatstroke is an *emergency.* You do not have time to wait for help. *Start treatment at once.* Evacuate after cooling. Damage to liver and kidneys may become apparent over the next few days.

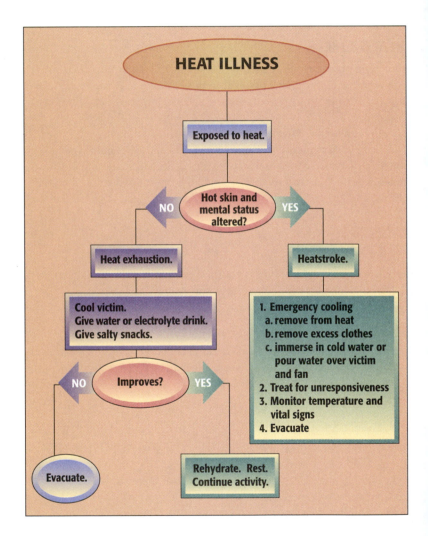

Fallacies about Heatstroke and Heat Illness

- The skin is always hot and dry.
- It takes several days of heat stress to develop.
- "Sport" drinks will keep your electrolytes normal.
- You should not drink too much water or your performance will suffer.
- You can train yourself to go with less water.
- Physical fitness prevents heat illness.

Heat Exhaustion vs. Heatstroke

TABLE 15.3

	Heat Exhaustion	Heatstroke
Mental state	Mild, brief confusion	Confusion progresses to coma, does not resolve quickly
Temperature	Normal to moderate elevation	Extreme elevation above 105°F (41°C)
Temperature regulation	Heat-regulating mechanisms intact; temperature will fall with rest in shade and intake of fluid	Heat-regulating mechanism fails and requires aggressive cooling measures
Skin	Often cool, clammy	Hot, may be moist or dry
Pulse	Mild elevation (100–120)	Markedly elevated (120–140), often weak
Injury to other organs	No underlying damage	May lead to liver, kidney damage
Evacuation	Treat in field; victim may continue activity when feeling better	Must evacuate rapidly for further treatment and monitoring

HEAT CRAMPS

Heat cramps occur alone or accompany heat exhaustion and are also caused by salt and water depletion during physical activity.

What to Look For

> ➤ cramps in the calf, thighs, or abdomen, usually beginning after exercise has stopped

What to Do

1. Stretch the affected muscles.

2. Give salted fluids; do *not* give salt tablets (unless 1–2 tablets dissolved in 1 qt. water)

Lightning Injury

The electric discharge of lightning during a thunderstorm is very powerful (30,000,000 volts and 250,000 amps), but very short-lived (1 to 100 milliseconds). Lightning kills by stopping the heart and breathing; external injury and both superficial and deep burns occur but are uncommon. There is little field management of lightning injuries. By the time the first-aider arrives on the scene, the damage has been done. General protection and support of the victim may be the most important first aid to be given.

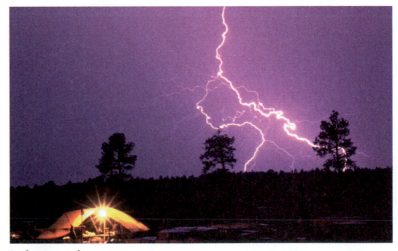

Lightning strike

During a thunderstorm, you should:

- Find shelter in a stone or brick building or a car (the metal body, not the rubber tires, affords protection).
- Squat on your heels to avoid being the highest object around and to keep ground currents from passing through your body.
- Stay in thick bush or among low trees, if in a forest.
- Separate from one another if in a group; remain 100 feet from the nearest person.
- Avoid metal conductors, such as ice axes.

Avoid

➤ isolated tall trees, hilltops, power lines or pylons, small exposed shelters

➤ tents, because the poles and wet fabric act as conductors

➤ hill ridges and summits (if unavoidable seek the lowest point)

➤ rock walls—stay 10 feet (3 m) away to avoid side flashes

➤ caves

TYPES OF INJURY

One-third of all people struck by lightning die. Some recover spontaneously and begin breathing within seconds.

What to Look For

➤ Loss of consciousness. Lightning may enter by the eyes (and cause later cataracts and blindness) or ears (rupturing the drum or mastoid and causing later deafness) and cause victims to lose consciousness. They may be confused after recovery.

➤ Superficial steam burns occur in moist areas in linear, rosettelike, or feathery patterns. Deep burns are rare. Clothing may be blasted apart and shredded.

➤ If the person is standing, the energy may flow up one leg and down the other, literally blowing the shoes and socks off.

➤ Blue, mottled limbs caused by intense blood vessel spasm.

➤ Intense generalized contraction of muscles may throw the person to the ground, fracturing bones or causing internal injury.

What to Do

1. Check ABCs. If the victim is still breathing and moaning he or she will probably recover.

2. Immediate CPR if the heart and breathing have stopped (see appendix A). Although many people have recovered after the heart has stopped, the outlook is poor but more favorable than in other types of cardiorespiratory arrest. Prolonged resuscitation is warranted, especially if the person can be taken to a facility with advanced life support (ALS).

3. If pulse is present, and there is no breathing, give rescue breaths as long as possible.

4. Check for injuries.

5. Give supportive care if the person survives; maintain airway, provide shelter, and monitor vital signs.

6. Evacuate. Don't be afraid to touch lightning victims; they do not store an electrical charge that can affect the rescuer.

Lightning Fallacies

- A lightning strike is always fatal.
- You cannot be hit if you have heard the thunder.
- Lightning only strikes during a storm.
- You are totally safe inside a building.
- If there is no external injury, there is no internal injury.
- Someone struck by lightning is dangerous to touch and is still "charged."
- If you are not killed by the lightning you will be OK.
- Lightning never strikes twice in the same place.

chapter 16

Poisons, Toxins, and Poisonous Plants

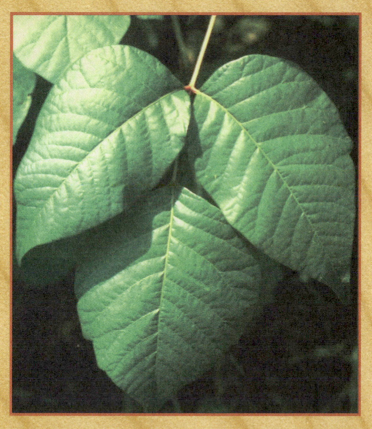

Carbon Monoxide Poisoning • Toxic Plants and Poisons •

Plant-Induced Dermatitis: Poison Ivy, Poison Oak,

and Poison Sumac

We are constantly encountering chemicals and plants whose toxic properties are unknown to us. Commonly used medications, pesticides, insect repellents, and sunscreens are all toxic to some people, even when used appropriately, and can be toxic to anyone if used inappropriately. The danger of misuse and overdosage is particularly likely in small children.

Chemical poisons are not common in the wilderness, and those most likely to be ingested will be medications. You cannot be expected to know the antidote to every chemical. Learn the simple principles used to treat most poisonings.

Few of us are expert in the identification of toxic plants and mushrooms: nettle stings may result in trivial irritation for a short time, while eating a dangerous mushroom may result in death. As in so many areas of wilderness first aid, some knowledge of what we may encounter—what is dangerous, what is safe—is extremely important. The safest policy is never to touch or eat a plant unless you know, with certainty, that it is safe.

Carbon Monoxide Poisoning

In the outdoors, the most likely cause of gas poisoning is carbon monoxide inhalation due to cooking on a stove in a tightly closed tent or snow cave, a camper with a faulty heater or stove, or prolonged use of a car heater with the motor idling while held up in a storm. Beware of the possible accumulation of a toxic gas as the cause of collapse in a confined space.

Victims of inhaled poisons are often unaware of the presence of a toxic gas, so it may be difficult to tell if someone has inhaled a toxic gas. The symptoms of inhaled poisons worsen or improve, depending on the proximity to the source (for gases); the closer to the source, the worse the symptoms.

What to Look For

➤ A complaint of "winter flu"—sometimes a symptom of carbon monoxide poisoning, but without low-grade fever, generalized aching, or swollen glands

➤ Similar symptoms in others exposed

➤ Sick pets

➤ Difficulty with breathing

➤ Headache

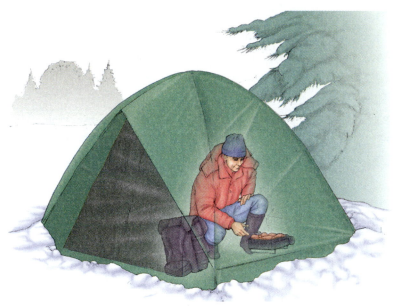

Cooking in a closed tent is dangerous and may lead to carbon monoxide poisoning.

➤ Ringing in the ears (tinnitus)

➤ Chest pain (angina)

➤ Muscle weakness

➤ Nausea and vomiting

➤ Dizziness and blurred or double vision

➤ Altered mental status

➤ Cardiac arrest

➤ In the terminal stages of carbon monoxide poisoning, bright-pink skin (as opposed to victims of other forms of asphyxia, in whom the skin will be bluish-gray)

What to Do

1. Do not move into an enclosed space where someone has already collapsed without first trying to determine the cause of the problem.

2. When the site is safe, move the victim into fresh air immediately.

3. Check ABCs.

4. Give oxygen, if available.

5. Call for rescue; evacuate as soon as possible.

Toxic Plants and Poisons

Fortunately, most poison ingestions happen with products or plants of low toxicity or with amounts so small that severe poisoning rarely occurs. However, the potential for severe or fatal poisoning is always present.

Swallowed poisons usually remain in the stomach only a short time, and the stomach absorbs only small amounts. Most absorption takes place after the poison passes into the small intestine.

Do not eat plants you cannot identify. Never eat mushrooms unless you are *absolutely certain* that they are safe. In the rare event that some-one in a wilderness setting far from the nearest medical help eats a potentially lethal mushroom, it may be necessary to induce vomiting. A teaspoonful of liquid soap in a cup of water may be the only agent available and is frequently effective.

What to Look For

➤ abdominal pain and cramping

➤ nausea or vomiting

➤ diarrhea

➤ burns, odor, stains around and in the mouth

➤ drowsiness or unconsciousness

➤ poison containers or evidence of poisonous plants nearby

What to Do

1. Determine critical information:
   - age and size of victim
   - what was swallowed (e.g., a "taste," a "handful")
   - how much was swallowed
   - when it was swallowed

2. Place the victim on the left side to position the end of the stomach where it enters the small intestine straight up. Gravity will delay by as much as 2 hours advancement of the poison into the small intestine. The side position also helps prevent inhalation into the lungs if vomiting occurs.

3. Evacuate as soon as possible.

4. If the poison is from a plant that you cannot identify, take a specimen for identification by an expert.

 ## DO NOT

- give strong salt solutions; this is dangerous, especially in children.
- induce vomiting in the following instances:
  - the victim swallowed a petroleum product (e.g., kerosene, gasoline, lighter fluid).
  - the victim is having seizures.
  - the victim is unconscious or drowsy.
  - the victim is in the third trimester (last three months) of pregnancy.
  - the victim is less than 6 months old.

The treatment of severe poisoning in the wilderness may be impossible because antidotes such as activated charcoal will never be available. Evacuate all victims of suspected poisoning, preferably to a hospital, as soon as possible.

Plant-Induced Dermatitis: Poison Ivy, Poison Oak, and Poison Sumac

Poison ivy, oak, and sumac are the three most common causes of contact dermatitis in the United States. Poison ivy occurs in every state except Hawaii and Alaska. It is the most widespread of the three. Poison oak occurs in two forms—Western and Southern. Sumac is found in the swamps of the East and South.

The cause of the allergy is contact with a resin, urushiol, in the plant stalk and leaves. During the winter the resin is still present in the stalk, but is not in the fallen leaves. Almost 50% of people in the United States are sensitive to the resin. The reaction develops within 8 to 48 hours after exposure, first as a line of small blisters where the skin brushed against the plant, followed by redness, swelling, and larger blisters. The blister fluid does not contain the irritant.

Resin can become attached to clothing and the fur of animals. A pet dog may be the source of contact. The resin can be spread soon after contact by the hands of the victim through scratching or during personal hygiene. Washing the hands after contact prevents further spread.

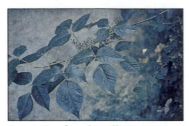

Poison ivy, found in all 48 contiguous U.S. states

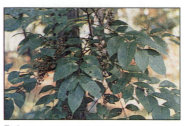

Poison sumac

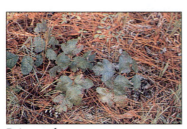

Poison oak

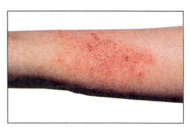

Poison ivy dermatitis

What to Look For

➤ itching, redness, swelling, and blisters on skin exposed to the resin

➤ reactions starting 8–48 hours after exposure. The reaction may continue to erupt in different areas for several days.

What to Do

1. Wash the exposed body parts thoroughly with cold water as soon as possible after known contact. The resin is firmly fixed to the skin within 30 minutes and cannot then be washed off except with special solutions (e.g., Technu Poison Oak-n-Ivy Cleaner™). Many victims are unaware of their contact until the itching and rash begin, several hours or days later.

2. For mild, localized contact, apply calamine lotion or hydrocortisone ointment or cream, 1.0%.

3. For a more severe, generalized eruption, apply calamine as an immediate treatment, but seek medical care for treatment with prescription steroids.

4. As a temporary measure, apply hydrocortisone ointment or cream (see appendix B), covered with a transparent plastic wrap and lightly bound with an elastic or self-adhering bandage.

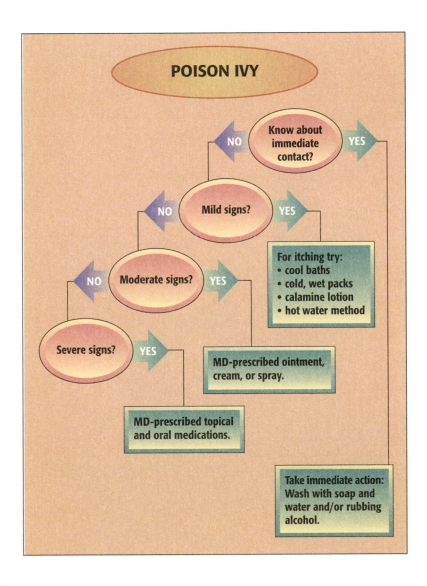

PREVENTION

- Learn to recognize the plants.
- After hiking through infested areas, wash hands, clothes, and any accompanying pets. Three barrier creams are useful for pre-exposure prevention: StokoGard Outdoor Cream™, Ivy Shield™, and Organoclay™.

Animal Bites, Human Bites, and Snakebites

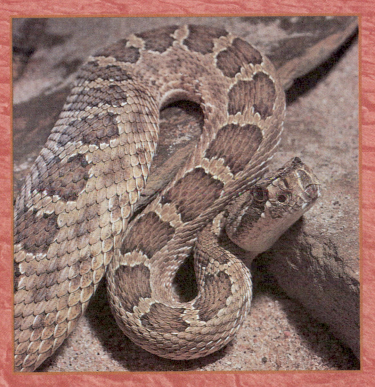

Animal Attacks • Human Bites • Snakebites

The wilderness traveler is sure to encounter animals; the species will depend on the geography. The animals will vary in size and ferocity, but it is not only the large and obviously aggressive that present danger. A small, rabid skunk is far more dangerous than a placid grizzly bear that turns and runs at the first sign of a human scent.

The first-aider should be aware of the animals likely to be seen, their appearance and identifying marks, their habits and habitats. An attacking animal may not remain in the area to be identified, and the victim may be too frightened to give a coherent account and description. If the animal is large and has horns or antlers, precise identification is not as important as the injuries suffered. If, however, the animal is potentially venomous, identification may be critical in deciding whether to evacuate the victim.

Animal Attacks

WILD ANIMALS

In Asia and Africa, attacks by elephants, hippos, lions, tigers, crocodiles, and snakes kill thousands of people every year. Snakebites alone cause 30,000 to 50,000 deaths per year in Asia, but fewer than 10 to 15 deaths per year in the United States.

In North America the wild animals most likely to attack humans are bears (both black and grizzly), bison, moose, cougars, and alligators. Not all injuries are bites. Severe injuries result from victims being thrown in the air, gored by antlers, butted, or trampled on the ground. Injuries include puncture wounds, bites, lacerations, bruises, fractures, rupture of internal organs, and evisceration. Many small animals such as squirrels and chipmunks bite people trying to feed them; these bites are seldom serious. (The dangers of infection and rabies are discussed below.)

DOMESTIC ANIMALS

Most animal bites in the United States are inflicted by dogs (2 million bites yearly) and by cats. Dog bites can be severe and sometimes lethal. The simple bites tend to be puncture wounds; more severe bites are tearing lacerations.

Cat bites should also be treated seriously. The fangs of a cat are short and sharp and inflict puncture wounds that frequently become infected. Most cat bites occur on the hands and may puncture tendons and joints.

What to Do

The principles of treatment are the same for injuries inflicted by domestic or wild animals.

1. If the wound is not bleeding heavily, irrigate it with water for 5 to 10 minutes (see page 64). Remove any foreign material. Only the superficial entrance of a puncture wound can be cleaned; extensive scrubbing cannot clean the depths of a puncture wound. Control bleeding with pressure (see pages 60–62 for details).

2. If there is a possibility of rabies, wash the wound with soap and water or with Zephiran™.

3. After a large animal attacks, examine the victim for internal injuries.

4. Cover wounds with a sterile dressing.

5. Evacuate the victim.

RABIES

Rabies is a fatal viral infection of the brain that may follow the bite of a rabid animal. The disease only affects warm-blooded animals.

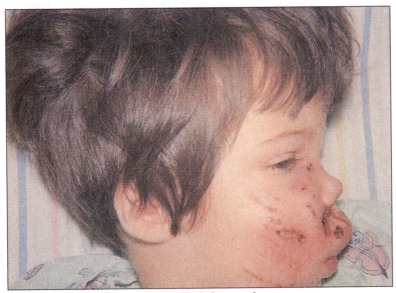

Dog bite, showing characteristic multiple bite marks

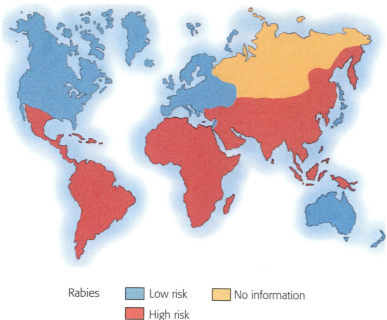

Rabies   ▢ Low risk   ▢ No information
          ▢ High risk

Most industrial, Western nations have effective control systems for domestic animals, but South and Central America, Africa, and Asia have poor controls and a high incidence of rabies in dogs. Some island countries, such as Britain and New Zealand, have eliminated rabies through strict quarantine regulations.

In North America, strict rabies control programs in domestic animals have made the disease rare. The reservoir of rabies in wild animals, however, remains large. Animals most commonly infected are skunks, raccoons, and bats. Foxes are occasionally found to be rabid, but rodents only rarely. In 1990 only 148 domestic dogs in the United States were found to be infected.

Rabies is found in all climes but not in all countries. There are thousands of cases per year in many countries, but in the United States there have been fewer than four human cases per year since 1980. All cases resulted from dog and bat bites, and the victims were mostly bitten outside the United States but developed rabies after returning home.

Consider rabies possible

- in an area or country where rabies is endemic
- if a bite by a dog, cat, skunk, raccoon, or fox is unprovoked and the skin is broken

- if bitten by a bat
- if bitten by a large carnivore
- if an already open wound or abrasion is licked by a potentially rabid animal

Rabies vaccines and serum are effective even if given after exposure. The sooner antirabies serum is given after a bite the better the chance of recovery. As there is no other treatment, the correct management after exposure is very important.

What to Do

1. The victim:
   - Wash the bite vigorously with a strong solution of soap and water or irrigate the bite marks with Zephiran™. Iodine solutions are not as effective, but in the absence of other agents use a diluted solution of Betadine™ (10% diluted to 1%).

2. The animal:

   The brain of an infected animal must be examined to make an exact diagnosis. Therefore it may be necessary to capture or kill the animal.
   - *Domestic animals:* Report the incident to the local health and animal control authorities. The animal will then be kept for 10 days to see if signs of rabies become obvious.
   - *Wild animals:* It may be difficult or impossible to capture a wild animal. Kill or capture the animal only if feasible without risk of being bitten. Deliver the body to the local health authority for diagnostic examination.

DO NOT
- try to capture the animal yourself.
- approach the animal.
- kill the animal unless it is wild and likely to escape. If it is killed, protect the head and brain from damage for examination for rabies. Transport the dead animal intact to prevent exposure to potentially infected tissues or saliva. Refrigerate, but do not freeze, animal remains.

<table>
<tr><td>**P R E V E N T I O N**</td><td>Preventive immunization is recommended for veterinarians, zoologists, and biologists who handle wild animals.

• Bats are a common reservoir of rabies. Spelunkers who explore caves heavily occupied by bats should be immunized.

• In countries where rabies is common, travelers should take great care in approaching village dogs or cats, monkeys, or any wild animals.</td></tr>
</table>

Human Bites

Any contact between the teeth and saliva of one human that causes an open wound on another is, technically, a bite (e.g., a hand injury caused by hitting another person's teeth during a fist fight is a bite). Wound infections are more common after human bites than animal bites.

What to Do

1. Wash the wound with soap and water for 5 to 10 minutes. Rinse liberally with water.
2. Control bleeding with pressure (see pages 60–62).
3. Cover with a sterile dressing.
4. Seek medical care and tetanus immunization, if needed.

Snakebites

This section deals only with snakes found in North America. Travelers to other areas should consult appropriate authorities for local information.

Only two snake families in the United States are poisonous: *pit vipers* (rattlesnakes, copperheads, and water moccasins) and *coral snakes.*

Pit vipers have a triangular, flat head, wider than the neck; vertical, elliptical pupils ("cat's eye"); and a heat-sensitive "pit" located between the eye and nostril.

The coral snake is small and very colorful, with a series of bright red, yellow, and black bands that go all the way around its body. Every alternate band is yellow, and the snout is black. The color banding is similar to that of the nonvenomous king snake, but when in doubt, remember: "Red on yellow, kill a fellow; red on black, venom lack."

The venom of young snakes is as toxic as that of adults, but the larger volume injected by adults usually causes a more severe reaction.

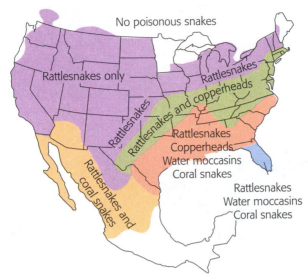

Distribution of poisonous snakes in the United States

PIT VIPER SNAKEBITE

Rattlesnakes inflict about 65 percent of all venomous snakebites and cause nearly all snakebite deaths in the United States. There are fewer than 15 snakebite deaths per year in the United States.

Twenty-five percent of rattlesnake bites are "dry"; no venom is injected. There may be a fang mark, but no local or systemic symptoms.

What to Look For

➤ severe burning pain at the bite site

➤ two small puncture wounds about ¼" to 1½" apart (some cases may have only one fang mark). If the snake has struck several times, there may be more than two fang marks.

➤ swelling, starting within 5 minutes and progressing up the extremity in the next hour. Swelling may continue to advance up the limb for several hours.

➤ discoloration and blood-filled blisters developing in 6 to 48 hours

➤ in severe cases: nausea, vomiting, sweating, weakness, bleeding, coma, and death

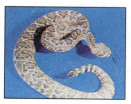

Rattlesnake

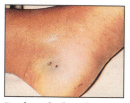

Rattlesnake bite (note two fang marks)

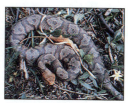

Copperhead snake

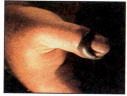

Copperhead bite two hours after bite

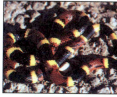

Coral snake, America's most venomous snake

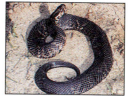

Watermoccasin (cottonmouth)

What to Do

Most snakebites happen within a few hours of a medical facility where antivenin is available. Bites without signs of venom injection require only a tetanus shot and care of the bite wounds.

1. Get the victim away from the snake. Snakes strike across a distance equal to half their body length and can bite more than once. Do not attempt to capture or kill the snake, and do not touch the head of an apparently dead snake: it may be able to bite reflexively for as long as an hour after "death."

2. Suction is only minimally effective and must be started within 2 to 3 minutes. Do not attempt oral suction or incising the skin. The Sawyer Extractor™ can remove up to 20%–30% of injected venom if applied within 2 to 3 minutes of the bite. No skin incision is necessary. If an Extractor is available, use it at once; but if none is available, do not waste time looking for one.

3. If there are immediate, severe symptoms, keep the victim quiet. Activity increases venom absorption. Send for help immediately.

4. To be effective, antivenin is best given within 4 to 6 hours after the bite. Start to evacuate all victims at once.

5. Use a sling or a splint to immobilize the limb loosely.

6. If there is no immediate reaction, start to walk slowly with the victim to the trailhead. Sending for help may take longer than walking out. If evacuation is prolonged and there are no symptoms after 6 to 8 hours, there has probably been no envenomation except in the case of coral snakebite.

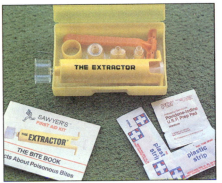

Extractor kit

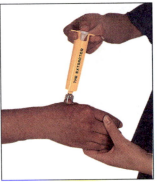

Strong suction raises skin and withdraws poison.

 DO NOT

- use cold or ice, which does not inactivate the venom and poses a frostbite hazard.
- use the "cut-and-suck" method, which can damage blood vessels and nerves.
- use mouth suction; your mouth is filled with bacteria, and you may infect the wound.
- use electric shock; no medical studies support this method.
- use a tourniquet, which can cause serious damage if wound too tight.
- use alcohol, which dilates vessels and compounds shock.
- use aspirin, which increases bleeding.

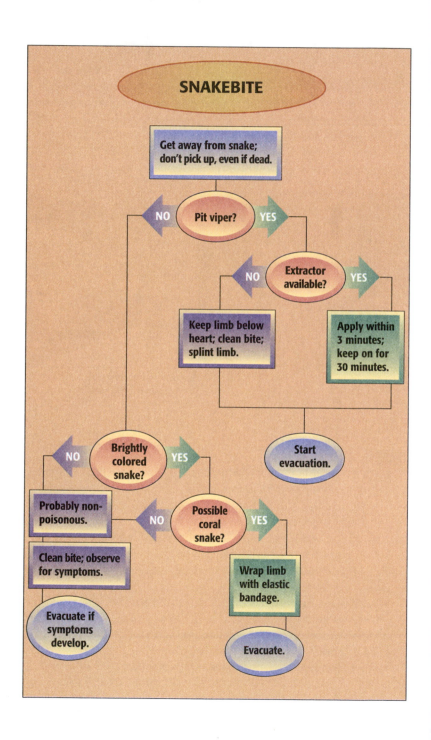

SNAKEBITE

Get away from snake; don't pick up, even if dead.

Pit viper? — NO / YES

Extractor available? — NO / YES

Keep limb below heart; clean bite; splint limb.

Apply within 3 minutes; keep on for 30 minutes.

Brightly colored snake? — NO / YES

Start evacuation.

Probably non-poisonous.

Possible coral snake? — NO / YES

Clean bite; observe for symptoms.

Wrap limb with elastic bandage.

Evacuate if symptoms develop.

Evacuate.

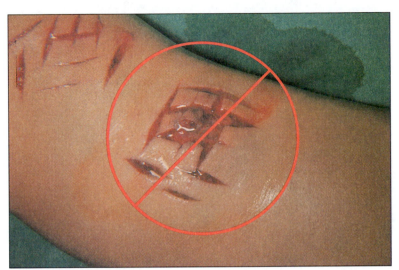

Do not incise a snakebite.

CORAL SNAKEBITE

The coral snake is America's most venomous snake, but it rarely bites humans. It is nocturnal and not aggressive. Its fangs are short, and it tends to hang on and "chew" venom into the victim rather than strike and release like a pit viper.

What to Look For

➤ Local, immediate signs are minimal. The absence of immediate symptoms is *not* evidence of a harmless bite. Several hours may pass before the onset of respiratory depression, double vision, or difficulty in swallowing.

What to Do

1. Keep the victim calm.
2. Clean the bite with soap and water.
3. Evacuate to hospital for antivenin.

NONPOISONOUS SNAKEBITE

Nonpoisonous snakes may leave toothmarks in a horseshoe shape on the victim's skin. There may be some swelling and tenderness but no evidence of significant envenomation.

What to Do

1. Clean the bite with soap and water.
2. Care for the bite as a minor wound.
3. Seek medical care; a tetanus booster may be needed.

PREVENTION

- Most snakes are nocturnal and hide from the heat in the middle of the day. At night, carry a flashlight and watch where you step.

- During the day do not step into places where you cannot see; do not reach up to ledges or put your hands down holes. Wear high boots. If you see a snake, do not try to catch or kill it. Stand still and let it move away.

- If someone has been bitten, try and get one good look at the snake, then leave it alone—avoid having two victims to evacuate.

CHAPTER 18

Insect and Arthropod Bites and Stings

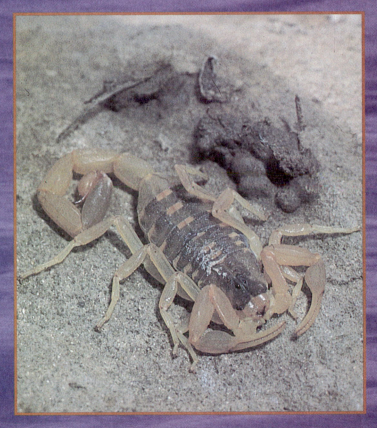

Spider Bites • Scorpion Stings • Centipede Bites •

Tick Bites • Insect Stings • Insect Repellents

Wilderness travelers generally worry about "bugs" and take precautions to avoid being bitten. Most bites and stings are merely annoying; others, such as the bites of some ticks and the sting of an Anopheles mosquito, may give rise to dangerous disease.

This chapter deals with the more common bites and stings that occur in North America and does not deal with the dozens of species in other countries around the world that give painful or sometimes lethal bites. Travelers going beyond North America should become familiar with the local insects and the diseases they carry. Information is available from state health departments or the Centers for Disease Control (see page 9).

Spider Bites

Many spiders are venomous, but few have either venom that is dangerous to humans or fangs long enough to penetrate human skin. Exceptions in North America include the black widow, brown recluse, hobo spider, and tarantula. Death from spider bite is rare in North America.

BLACK WIDOW SPIDER

The black widow spider is found throughout the world. Only the female is dangerous; she has a glossy black body with a red spot (often in the shape of an hourglass) on the abdomen. Identification of a black widow spider bite is difficult because most likely the spider will not be seen.

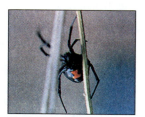

Black widow spider

What to Look For

➤ a sharp pinprick may be felt, although some victims are unaware of being bitten; no mark may be visible

➤ faint red bite marks, which appear later

➤ muscle stiffness and cramps, affecting the bitten limb and ascending to the abdomen and thorax

➤ headache, chills, fever, heavy sweating, dizziness, nausea, vomiting, and severe abdominal pain occurring later

What to Do

1. If possible, catch the spider for identification. Save the body, even if it is crushed.
2. Clean the bitten area with soap and water.

3. Relieve pain, which may be severe, with an ice pack on the bite. Administer pain medication orally.

4. Check the ABCs.

5. Seek medical attention immediately. Antivenin is available but is usually given only to children, the elderly, those with high blood pressure, pregnant women, or after severe envenomation.

BROWN RECLUSE SPIDER

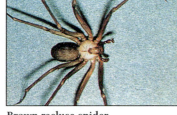

The brown recluse is a nondescript spider with a brown, sometimes purplish, violin-shaped figure on its back. It is generally found in the southern United States but has been identified as far north as Wisconsin.

Brown recluse spider

The brown northwestern hobo spider can be mistaken for the brown recluse; it is similar in appearance but does not have a "violin" marking. Its bite can be painful but not as dangerous as that of the brown recluse. The two spiders are found in widely separate geographic locations. Find out which spiders are located in your travel area. The brown recluse should not be implicated just from an initial skin lesion. Other spiders and even some insect bites can result in a large area of redness with a central blister or small ulcer.

What to Look For

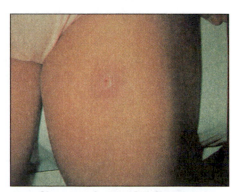

➤ during the early stages, a bite with a bull's-eye appearance—a central white core surrounded by red, ringed by a whitish or blue border. A blister at the site, along with redness and swelling, appears several hours after the bite.

Bite of brown recluse spider showing target pattern

➤ local pain, which may remain mild but can become severe. It then subsides, to be replaced by aching and itching.

➤ fever, weakness, vomiting, joint pain, and a rash

What to Do

1. Clean the bite with soap and water.

2. Relieve pain with an ice pack on the bite; give pain medication.

3. There is no immediate danger. Later, large areas of inflammation may develop. If this happens, seek medical attention promptly.

4. Capture or kill the spider for identification.

TARANTULA

The North American variety of this large, hairy spider has a frightening appearance but is almost always harmless. There is moderate pain at the bite but few later symptoms. In some areas other than North America, tarantulas are dangerous. Know the local species.

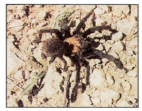
Tarantula

What to Do

1. Clean the bite with soap and water.

2. Relieve pain with an ice pack.

3. Evacuate the victim if the species is known to be dangerous.

Scorpion Stings

Scorpions are found worldwide in desert and semiarid regions. Dangerous species exist in both hemispheres In the southwestern United States, the bark scorpion is potentially lethal to small children and the elderly in poor health. Be aware of its appearance and distribution.

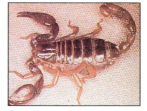
Scorpion

Scorpions look like miniature lobsters; they have pincers and a long upturned tail with a poisonous stinger. The sting causes immediate local pain and burning, followed by numbness or tingling. Symptoms include paralysis, muscle spasms, or breathing difficulties.

What to Look For

➤ instant local pain and burning (all bites)

➤ blurred vision, difficulty swallowing, slurred speech, numbness and tingling, occasional paralysis, muscle spasms, and breathing difficulties (severe bites)

➤ jerking and twitching (similar to a seizure)
➤ more severe symptoms in children than adults

What to Do

1. Check the ABCs.
2. Clean the bite site with soap and water.
3. Put an ice pack on the sting to relieve pain.
4. Evacuate the victim as soon as possible. Antivenin for bark scorpion bite is available only in Arizona. It is used only for severe envenomation in small children and the elderly.

Centipede Bites

Centipedes have small fangs and venom glands. If the fangs are long enough to penetrate skin there can be local envenomation. Burning pain, swelling, and redness may last up to three weeks.

What to Do

1. Most bites will get better without treatment. If symptoms persist, try administering antihistamines by mouth or applying hydrocortisone ointment on the bite.

Tick Bites

Tick bites are painless, and a tick can remain attached for days without the victim being aware of its presence. Some ticks can transmit serious diseases (including Lyme disease, Rocky Mountain spotted fever, and tick paralysis), but most tick bites are harmless.

 DO NOT

- **use petroleum jelly, fingernail polish, rubbing alcohol, a hot match, petroleum products, or gasoline to remove ticks. They are ineffective.**

What to Do

Ticks are difficult to remove because they secrete a cement that anchors them to the skin. Improper or partial removal can lead to local infection.

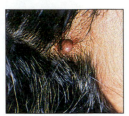

Tick embedded and engorged with victim's blood

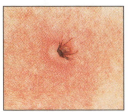

Tick embedded

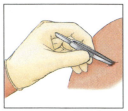

Removing a tick with tweezers

1. Remove the tick using one of these methods:
   - tweezers (specially designed tweezers are available)
   - fingers (protect your skin with paper or gloves)
2. Grasp the tick close to the skin surface and pull steadily; or lift the tick slightly upward, then pull parallel to the skin until the tick detaches. If the head is still embedded in the skin, remove it with a needle as you would a splinter.
3. Wash the bite with soap and water.
4. If removal of the tick was painful, put an ice pack on the bite.
5. Watch for signs of local infection or unexplained symptoms of tick-borne illness (severe headache, fever, or rash) appearing 3 to 30 days after discovery of the tick. If symptoms appear, seek medical attention immediately.

 DO NOT
   - grab the rear of the tick; the gut may rupture and the contents be squeezed out, causing infection.
   - twist or jerk the tick. This may cause incomplete removal.

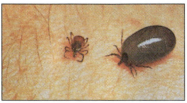

Deer ticks: not engorged and blood engorged

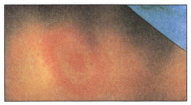

Lyme disease rash

LYME DISEASE

Lyme disease, a potentially serious tick-borne infection, affects the joints, skin, heart, and nervous system. The disease is caused by a corkscrew-shaped bacterium, or spirochaete, that is transported by ticks from deer and mice to humans. In the northeastern United States, the deer tick is the main carrier; in the west it is the black-legged tick.

Most infections are transmitted by the nymph form of the tick, which is about as big as a period (.) and difficult to see. Only 20% of infections are transmitted by adult ticks. The tick may have to be attached for 24 hours before transmitting infection; the longer a tick is attached, the greater the chance of infection.

Most victims of Lyme disease do not remember being bitten by a tick, because the disease may not become manifest until several weeks after the victim returns home.

What to Look For

➤ in early stages: distinctive rash (3 days to 1 month), fatigue, fever, chills, weakness, headaches, stiff necks, muscle or joint pains

➤ in later stages: one-sided paralysis, arthritis, meningitis, nerve or heart damage

What to Do

1. If any symptoms develop within a month of a tick bite, consult a doctor. Antibiotic treatment is usually curative, but is not necessary after every tick bite.

PREVENTION
- Wear long trousers tucked into socks during early summer tick season and when walking through long grass and infested areas.
- Spray clothing with permethrin insect repellent (see page 278).
- After hiking in tick-infested areas, inspect the *whole* body for ticks.

Insect Stings

More people die every year in the United States from bee, hornet, and wasp stings than from snakebites. The common stinging insects are the honeybee, bumblebee, yellow jacket, wasp, and fire ant. A single sting to a severely allergic person may be fatal within minutes to an hour. Many people who die have had no previous history of severe reactions to stings. Multiple stings can kill, whether or not the person is allergic to stinging insects. Massive, multiple stings are rare, but with the entrance into the United States of Africanized "killer" bees from South and Central America, multiple-sting cases are likely to increase. The venom of these bees is no more potent than that of the European type; however, killer bees earned their nickname with their aggressiveness and swarming attacks.

What to Look For

The sooner after the sting symptoms develop, the more serious the reaction.

➤ *local reactions:* brief pain, redness and swelling around the sting site, itching, and heat

➤ *generalized reactions:* diffuse skin redness, hives, localized swelling of lips or tongue, "tickle" in throat, wheezing, abdominal cramps, diarrhea

➤ *life-threatening reactions:* inability to breathe due to swelling of the air passages and throat, bluish or gray skin color, seizures, unconsciousness

➤ The responses of victims vary. One sting is not necessarily equivalent to another, even within the same species, because the amount of venom injected varies from sting to sting.

➤ Stings to the mouth or eyes are more dangerous than stings to other body areas. The most dangerous stings in nonallergic individuals are those inside the throat, from accidentally swallowing an insect. Swelling in the airway—though not an allergic reaction—can cause serious obstruction to breathing.

What to Do

1. Look for a stinger embedded in the skin (Only the honeybee leaves its stinger embedded.) Stingers, unless removed, can continue to inject venom for 2 or 3 minutes. Scrape the stinger and venom sac off the skin with a knife blade, but avoid pressing on them.

 DO NOT

- pull the stinger with tweezers or fingers because you may squeeze more venom into the victim from the attached venom site.

2. Wash the sting site with soap and water.

3. Apply cold to the sting site for 15 to 20 minutes to relieve pain.

4. To relieve pain and itching, give a mild analgesic (e.g., aceta-minophen, ibuprofen) or use a topical medication such as Secta Sooth Sting Relief Swab™ or Sting Eze™. Hydrocortisone cream and antihistamine pills reduce local symptoms.

5. Observe victims for at least 60 minutes for signs of a serious allergic reaction (see chapter 13).

6. A large local reaction does not require epinephrine and does not indicate a risk of serious reaction after future stings. If the victim develops hives or redness and swelling all over the body and difficulty breathing, immediately administer epinephrine if available.

P R E V E N T I O N
   Do not approach or disturb wasp, bee, and ant nests. Do not walk in grass with bare feet. Choose campsites with care.
   Those who have had a serious reaction to an insect sting should carry with them at all times a kit with self-injectable epinephrine and should wear a medical alert bracelet/necklace identifying them as allergic to insect stings and should see an allergist for desensitization.

LICE

Lice are small parasites that live on clothes, hair, or skin and drink blood. There are three types: head lice, pubic lice, and body lice. Body lice live on clothing, while head lice and pubic lice attach themselves to the hair shafts. All cause itching.

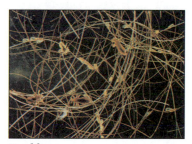

Head lice

   Lice are passed from person to person by direct contact or through clothes, bedding, hats, or hairbrushes. Pubic lice are most likely passed by sexual contact. Head lice are very common among schoolchildren. Body lice usually accompany poor hygiene. Lice do not live outdoors in the wild, and lice discovered on a trip usually would have been brought from home or picked up in a dwelling. Lice live only 2 to 3 weeks off the body on clothes and sleeping bags.

What to Do

1. Treat with nonprescription lice shampoo or lotion containing permethrin (Nix™), pyrethrins with peperonyl butoxide (RID™), or lindane (Kwell™).

2. Wash clothes, sleeping bags, pillowcases, or other bedding in hot water.

3. Do not share clothes or hairbrushes.

Insect Repellents

Chemical repellents include natural repellents (citronella, lemon eucalyptus); synthetic repellents (DEET, dimethylthalate); and insecticides (permethrin, deltamethrin, alphamethrin).

Citronella (Avon Skin-So-Soft™) and lemon eucalyptus provide 1 to 2 hours of protection. They are safe but not very effective and not recommended where serious protection is needed.

DEET (diethylmetatoluamide) is the most widely used repellent. Allergic reactions can occur when DEET is applied to the skin in high concentrations; it should not be used in concentrations greater than 35%. Although higher concentrations provide longer protection, new formulations have prolonged effect at lower concentrations. Some of the chemical is absorbed through the skin, and toxic reactions have been reported in small children. To avoid toxic effects, avoid the lips, eyes, and broken skin. Do not use DEET on infants. In children, especially, use low concentrations (10%) applied more frequently rather than high concentrations applied infrequently. DEET can be applied to clothing but may damage some synthetics, including polyesters.

Permethrin is an effective repellent against ticks, chiggers, mosquitoes, fleas, and sand flies. It should be applied only to clothing, not to the skin. Clothing, sleeping nets, or tents can be impregnated with permethrin by spraying or soaking in a solution. It does not stain, discolor, or degrade fabrics or plastics and maintains effectiveness on fabrics for weeks to months, even persisting through multiple washings.

In areas with mosquito-borne diseases, a permethrin-impregnated sleeping net is important protection. In addition, the traveler should wear long-sleeved shirts and long pants during dusk and dawn, when mosquitoes are most active. The combination of DEET on skin and permethrin on clothing provides maximum protection.

chapter 19

Water Emergencies

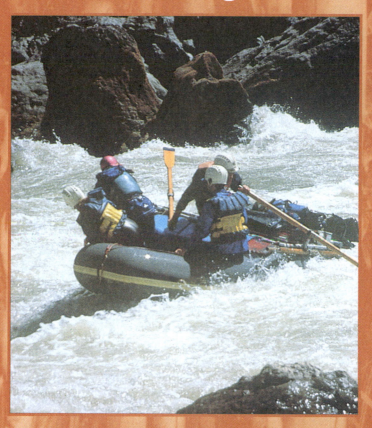

Submersion Incidents • Scuba Diving Injuries •

Marine Animal Stings

Submersion Incidents

A submersion incident is any medical condition caused by an underwater accident. *Drowning* means the victim is dead; a *near-drowning* victim survives at least 24 hours. There are no significant differences in mortality and physiological changes between victims who drown in fresh or salt water.

> **PREVENTION**
> Most submersion incidents are preventable. Learning to swim at a young age, close observation of toddlers around water, and minimizing drug and alcohol use around water would prevent the majority of accidents. For wilderness trips, general safety precautions, setting up of safety lines when crossing streams, and knowing the limits of your team and the hazards of the environment will help you minimize the risk of submersion incidents.

What to Look For

➤ The victim is seen struggling in the water, floating motionless, or lying at the bottom of a pool.

What to Do

The essentials of first aid for any water emergency are a safe rescue, application of the ABCs, and transport to the nearest medical facility.

1. Assess your resources and abilities before attempting rescue. Rescue of a submerged, drowned, or drowning victim may be dangerous.

2. Rescue the victim. Remember, *do not become a victim yourself!* The following guidelines are suggested for getting a victim safely out of the water: Reach, Throw, Row, Go (see page 281).

3. Treat the victim.
   - If unresponsive, check ABCs.
   - Begin rescue breathing and CPR if the victim is not breathing or is pulseless (see chapter 3).
   - If it is impossible to breathe for the victim, first try a finger sweep of the mouth and back of the throat to dislodge food, gum, or other foreign material obstructing the airway.
   - If this does not open the airway, try the Heimlich maneuver.
   - Protect the cervical spine in unresponsive victims and in victims of diving and/or surfing accidents or high falls.

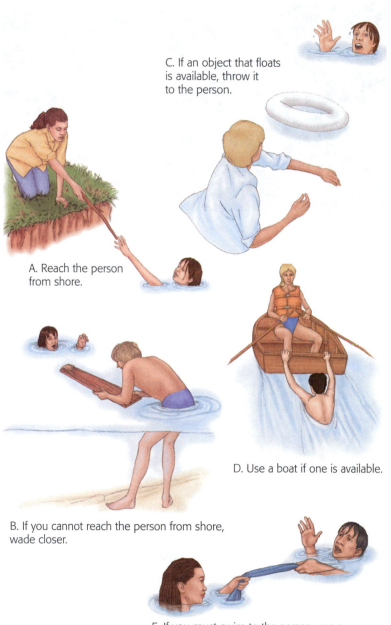

C. If an object that floats is available, throw it to the person.

A. Reach the person from shore.

B. If you cannot reach the person from shore, wade closer.

D. Use a boat if one is available.

E. If you must swim to the person, use a towel or board for him or her to hold onto. Do not let the person grab you.

Reach–Throw–Row–Go

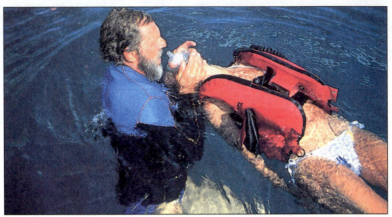

Stabilize cervical spine

4. Perform resuscitation (see chapter 3).
   • You need not start resuscitation if an adult is known to have been submerged more than 60 minutes in warm water.
   • Stop resuscitation after 30 minutes if there are no signs of life, unless the victim has been submerged in very cold water.
   • If submersion has been in very cold water, continue for at least 60 minutes with concurrent attempts to warm the victim.
   • If there is a heartbeat or a pulse, continue rescue breathing until spontaneous respirations resume or as long as possible.

5. Evacuate all victims who have been resuscitated. Assess the situation. Outside assistance may be required to transport the victim safely to the nearest medical facility or higher level of care. Think about your resources and the best way to handle the situation while minimizing further risk to other members of the rescue team.

6. Victims not requiring resuscitation, and whose only initial symptoms have been coughing or vomiting, require close observation but not immediate evacuation; evacuate for medical evaluation if cough or shortness of breath increases.

REMEMBER: Immediate treatment by ventilation at the scene is the most important factor in determining survival.

Scuba Diving Injuries

Scuba (self-contained underwater breathing apparatus) divers should be familiar with the medical problems of diving from their certified training course. Those who do not dive should understand the basic problems that divers may face and know how to begin appropriate treatment. Only pressure-related disorders will be discussed here.

As a diver descends, water pressure on the body increases. For each 33 feet of descent, the pressure increases by one atmosphere (1 atmosphere = 14.7 pounds per square inch): sea level = 1 atm; 33 feet = 2 atm; 66 feet = 3 atm.

This changing pressure is exerted over the entire body, but is only a problem for the gas-containing areas of the body (lungs, ears, sinuses), where changes in pressure create changes in gas volume. Increasing pressure during descent results in a decrease in gas volume, which reexpands on ascent. If gas pressure cannot equilibrate in a closed space, the vacuum effect on descent or the expansion during ascent may cause pain, rupture of blood vessels, or rupture of the weakest part of the enclosed space, such as the eardrum or air sacs of the lung. Illnesses and injuries due to the mechanical effects of pressure changes are called *dysbarism*.

Potential Problems Associated with Scuba Diving

Dysbarism
- barotrauma
- air embolism
- decompression sickness

Breathing-gas Problems
- nitrogen narcosis
- oxygen toxicity
- hypoxia
- carbon monoxide poisoning

Hazardous Marine Life

Environmental Problems
- motion sickness
- near-drowning
- hypothermia
- heat illness
- sunburn

Miscellaneous Problems
- hyperventilation
- panic/anxiety

DECOMPRESSION ILLNESS

The most serious medical problems arising from scuba diving are caused by gas bubbles forming in the tissues or entering the blood stream and lodging in the small vessels of the joints, spinal cord, brain, and other parts of the body. One source of gas bubbles is arterial gas embolism, or rupture of the small air sacs in the lung during rapid ascent. The other source is from generalized decompression.

Air contains about 20% oxygen and 80% nitrogen. Oxygen is consumed as a fuel by the body, but nitrogen, an inert gas, is not used and builds up under increasing pressure in the blood and tissues.

The nitrogen must be expelled through the lungs. As the pressure is reduced during ascent, if nitrogen accumulation exceeds its solubility, it will form gas bubbles. Divers must monitor their total time underwater at the maximum depth and adhere to precise schedules to assure that they will not stay down too long and accumulate too much nitrogen. If gas bubbles form, they may lodge in the small vessels of many different organs, disrupting circulation and causing serious problems.

ARTERIAL GAS EMBOLISM (AGE)

AGE develops within 5 minutes of surfacing.

What to Look For

➤ unconsciousness
➤ paralysis or weakness
➤ convulsions
➤ respiratory arrest
➤ dizziness or visual problems

DECOMPRESSION SICKNESS (DCS)

DCS develops after surfacing or may be delayed hours to days.

What to Look For

➤ joint or limb pain
➤ paralysis
➤ fatigue and weakness
➤ breathing difficulty
➤ numbness or tingling
➤ rash

What to Do

Regardless of the cause, most diving injuries can be treated initially with similar measures.

1. Evaluate ABCs, resuscitate as needed. Barotrauma may have caused near-drowning.

2. Give 100% oxygen. Early administration of 100% oxygen is very important. If no oxygen is available, contact the local EMS as soon as possible.

3. Place victim in the recovery position.

4. If victim is conscious and alert, give sips of water—no alcohol.

5. Protect victim from excessive cold and heat.

6. If a seizure occurs, prevent injury and maintain the airway. Continue giving 100% oxygen (see chapter 3).

7. Evaluate for other injuries, minor barotrauma problems, or environmental problems such as hypothermia.

8. Do neurologic examination (see page 286).

9. Contact the local EMS.

10. Get the victim with decompression sickness to recompression therapy in a hyperbaric (pressurized) chamber.

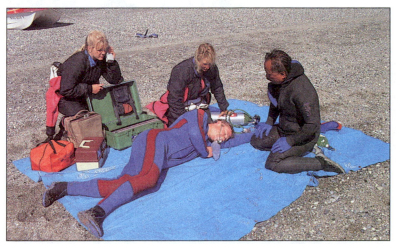

Recovery position: lateral recumbent (preferred) or supine (on back)

Neurologic Examination

1. Is the diver oriented to person, place, time?
2. Eyes: normal vision and movement, pupils equal? Any jerking motion?
3. Face: able to smile, grit teeth, whistle? Is sensation normal?
4. Hearing: normal?
5. Able to swallow?
6. Able to move tongue in all directions?
7. General muscle strength: weak? Equal on both sides?
8. Sensory: normal on both sides? Any numbness or complaints of tingling?
9. Balance and coordination: Can walk normally? Can walk a straight line? Can victim stand with feet together and close eyes with outstretched arms without falling over? Can victim accurately touch fingertip to nose?

What to Do

1. Establish/maintain airway.
2. Rescue breathing.
3. Contact local EMS.
4. CPR, if necessary.
5. 100% oxygen.
6. Place diver in supine or lateral recumbent position.
7. Give water if conscious and alert.

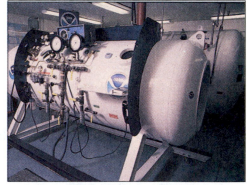

Hyperbaric chamber for recompression therapy

8. Contact DAN (Divers Alert Network)—1-919-684-8111 (24-hour diving emergencies).

Marine Animal Stings

PORTUGUESE MAN-OF-WAR, JELLYFISH, SEA ANEMONE

The Portuguese man-of-war and the jellyfish are two members of a large group of sea animals—coelenterates—with tentacles containing stinging

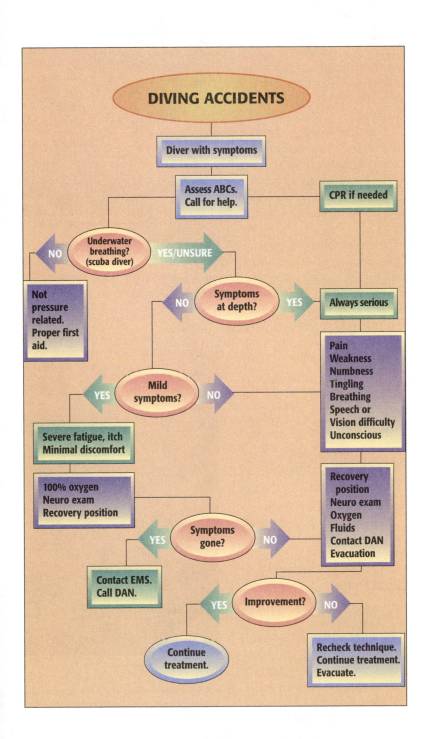

DIVING ACCIDENTS

Diver with symptoms

Assess ABCs. Call for help. — CPR if needed

Underwater breathing? (scuba diver) — NO / YES/UNSURE

Not pressure related. Proper first aid.

Symptoms at depth? — NO / YES — Always serious

Mild symptoms? — YES / NO

Pain
Weakness
Numbness
Tingling
Breathing
Speech or
Vision difficulty
Unconscious

Severe fatigue, itch
Minimal discomfort

100% oxygen
Neuro exam
Recovery position

Recovery position
Neuro exam
Oxygen
Fluids
Contact DAN
Evacuation

Symptoms gone? — YES / NO

Contact EMS. Call DAN.

Improvement? — YES / NO

Continue treatment.

Recheck technique. Continue treatment. Evacuate.

organs called nematocysts. Swimmers and divers who brush against nematocysts can receive serious, painful injuries. When washed ashore or onto rocks, dead jellyfish or tentacle fragments can still sting for a long time.

Reactions to stings vary from mild to severe. Most victims recover without medical attention; some need it immediately.

Portuguese man-of-war stings cause well-defined, whiplike welts or scattered red blotches, which usually disappear within 24 hours.

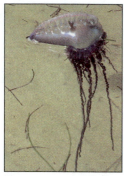

Portuguese man-of-war

Jellyfish stings cause burning pain that lasts half an hour, severe muscle cramping, and multiple thin lines of zigzag welts that may disappear within a few hours.

The severity of the reaction depends on the species, the number of nematocysts triggered, the age and health of the victim, and the extent of contact.

What to Look For

➤ pain, varying in severity

➤ whiplike streaks on the skin

➤ blisters, welts, scattered red blotches within 24 hours

➤ in more severe cases, headache, dizziness, paralysis, anaphylaxis

➤ possible coelenterate poisoning in all cases of unexplained collapse in ocean swimmers

What to Do

1. Immediately rinse with seawater (*not* fresh water, which causes nematocysts to activate); remove tentacles with tweezers. Do not touch tentacles with the bare hand.

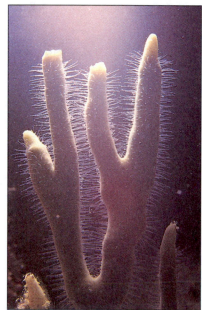

Fire coral is in the same family as Portuguese man-of-war. It has tiny nematocyst-bearing tentacles on the surface that cause the sting.

2. Apply vinegar, rubbing alcohol, or household ammonia (in order of preference) for 30 minutes or until pain is relieved.

3. After soaking with vinegar or alcohol, apply shaving cream or baking soda paste and shave the area to remove the nematocysts. Reapply vinegar or alcohol and soak for another 15 minutes.

4. Apply hydrocortisone cream (1%), antihistamine cream, or anesthetic ointment twice a day.

 DO NOT
- **rinse with fresh water or apply ice to the skin**
- **rub off the tentacles from the victim's skin—this activates the stinging cells.**

OTHER MARINE LIFE

Sting rays, sea urchins, catfish, stonefish, and scorpion fish are found in temperate, subtropical, and tropical waters, generally in shallow, sheltered bays. When a person steps on a ray, the tail whips up and the stinging organ is thrust into the foot. The large tail barb can also cause a severe laceration; the venom causes intense burning pain at the site, and pieces of the sting may remain in the wound.

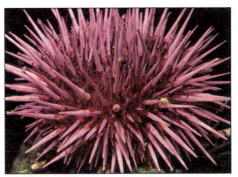

Sea urchin. Fish, ray, and urchin wounds may require exploration of the wound for embedded pieces of the spine.

What to Do

1. Irrigate the injured part with water immediately to remove venom and relieve pain; soak in hot water for 30 to 90 minutes. The water must be as hot as victim can tolerate.

2. Remove obvious pieces of the barb.

3. Treat as a puncture wound (see pages 62–64).

4. Seek medical attention promptly. Pieces of spine may be embedded in the wound. Consider a tetanus booster.

APPENDIX A

Essentials of Resuscitation

To obtain the skills necessary to resuscitate a person who has stopped breathing or is without circulation, we recommend that you take a course in cardiopulmonary resuscitation and basic life support given by the National Safety Council, the American Red Cross, or the American Heart Association. This chapter will provide you only with the essentials required to start resuscitation until someone with more skill takes over or the situation becomes obviously hopeless.

Basic Life Support

Basic life support (BLS) refers to lifesaving procedures that focus on the victim's airway, breathing, and circulation. BLS includes rescue breathing, cardiopulmonary resuscitation (CPR), and obstructed airway management.

Basic life support is effective only if started quickly, given skillfully, and followed by advanced life support, which includes electrical defibrillation of the heart. In the wilderness the chances of success with BLS alone are slight. You should therefore face the fact that few victims who require BLS in the wilderness will survive. But, in spite of that, you should be prepared to start BLS when necessary.

Resuscitation has two parts: rescue breathing (artificial respiration) and chest compression. Both together constitute cardiopulmonary resuscitation. Not everyone requires CPR; some victims require only rescue breathing.

What to Look For

➤ Open the airway and check for breathing (see chapter 3).

➤ Check the circulation (see chapter 3).

➤ Confirm that the victim is not breathing, has no pulse, and is motionless and unresponsive (otherwise recheck for breathing and pulse).

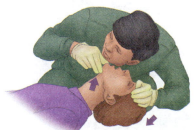

Listen and feel for movement of air, and look for rise and fall of chest. Open the airway with the head-tilt/chin-lift technique or with the jaw-thrust technique.

WHEN TO START CPR

Start CPR on a motionless person in whom it is known that respiration or circulation has stopped. If the person is hypothermic the delay in starting can be considerably longer, depending on the temperature of the victim (see chapter 3).

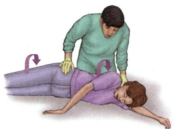

Gently roll victim's head and body together into face-up position.

What to Do

1. Logroll the victim onto his or her back.

2. Use the head-tilt/chin-lift method to open the airway.

3. Check for breathing.
   - *If breathing* and spinal injury is not suspected, place the victim in the recovery position.
   - If not breathing, give 2 slow breaths. If breaths go in, go to step 4.

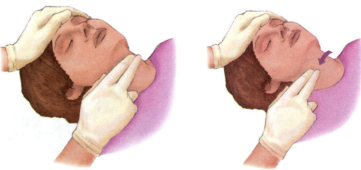

Check carotid pulse in groove next to Adam's apple.

- *If first breath unsuccessful,* retilt head and try another breath.
- *If still unsuccessful,* treat as for foreign body obstruction (see pages 296–297 for details of techniques).

4. Check pulse (carotid artery).
   - If there is a pulse, but no breathing, give rescue breaths (1 breath every 5 seconds).
   - If there is no pulse, give CPR (cycles of 15 chest compressions followed by 2 breaths).

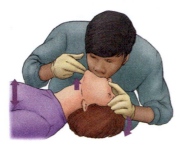

Technique of rescue breathing

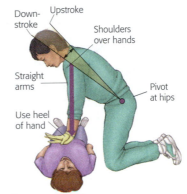

Down-stroke   Upstroke

Shoulders over hands

Straight arms

Pivot at hips

Use heel of hand

Technique of CPR

5. If help is available, assign one person to provide rescue breaths and you or another to do the cardiac compression at a rate of 5 compressions to one breath. Check the pulse every minute.

6. Continue resuscitation until more skilled rescuers can take over, you are exhausted, efforts are still unsuccessful after 30 minutes, the victim has been pronounced dead by a medical doctor, or it is obvious that the victim has died.

WHEN TO GIVE PROLONGED CPR

- The victim is hypothermic with a compressible chest.
- The victim has been submersed in cold water.
- There is cardiac arrest due to lightning or electric shock.

WHEN NOT TO START CPR

- The victim has a lethal injury—severe head injury, massive chest injury, etc.

TABLE A.1

**Chances of Survival
(Survival Rate %)**

		Time Until Advanced Cardiac Life Support Begins		
		<8 min.	8–16 min.	>16 min.
Time Until Basic Life Support (CPR)	<4 min.	43%	19%	10%
	4–8 min.	27%	19%	6%
	>8 min.	N/A	7%	0%

Source: National Ski Patrol, based upon Eisenberg, et. al., *JAMA,* 1979; 241:1905–1907.

- There are signs that the victim has been dead for some time—rigor mortis, lividity (the purple color of blood as it sinks to the lowest part of a corpse).
- The known time from incident to resuscitation is too great for success—e.g., 15 minutes since cardiac arrest; more than 1 hour of submersion of an adult in water.
- The victim is in cardiac arrest following severe trauma.
- The victim is hypothermic with a frozen, incompressible chest.
- The environment is unsafe and dangerous to the rescuers.

WHEN TO STOP CPR

- The victim revives.
- Another trained rescuer takes over.
- You are too exhausted to continue.
- The situation becomes unsafe for rescuers.
- A physician tells you to stop.
- CPR has been given for 30 minutes without signs of recovery, except when there are indications for prolonged CPR (see above).

Children and Infants

The most likely wilderness accidents requiring the resuscitation of a child are drowning, a lightning strike, or severe trauma such as a head injury. Under all these circumstances the most important treatment is rescue breathing. The most common cause for cardiac arrest in a child is a primary respiratory arrest leading to lack of oxygen to the heart. Often, a child's resilient heart will restart with oxygen supplied by rescue breathing.

What to Do

1. Open airway.
2. Check for breathing.
   - *If not breathing*, give 2 slow breaths. If breaths go in, go to step 3.
   - *If first breath did not go in*, retilt head and give another.
   - *If still unsuccessful*, use adult foreign body obstruction procedures on pages 297–298 if a child. If an infant, see pages 298–300.
3. Check pulse (carotid for child and brachial for infant).
   - *If there is a pulse, but no breathing*, give rescue breaths (1 every 3 seconds).
   - If there is no pulse, give CPR (cycles of 5 chest compressions followed by 1 breath).

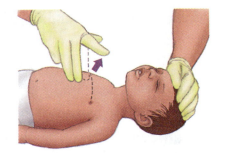

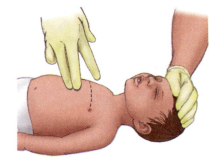

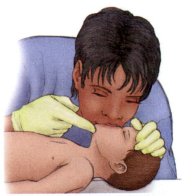

Use two fingers for chest compressions on an infant (use the heel of one hand for chest compressions on a child). Give CPR to infant with your mouth over both the victim's mouth and nose.

The principles of children's CPR are the same as for adults, *except*:

- Use only 1 hand on a child; use 2 fingertips on an infant.
- Compress at the rate of 100 per minute.
- Cover the infant's nose and mouth with your mouth, or mask for rescue breathing.
- Give 1 breath every 3 seconds or every 5 chest compressions.
- Check pulse every 10 cycles.
- Feel an infant's brachial pulse on inside of upper arm.

Airway Obstruction and Choking

Choking victims vary as to whether the victim (1) is conscious and has a partial airway obstruction, (2) is conscious and has a complete airway obstruction, (3) becomes unconscious as a result of complete airway obstruction, or (4) is found unconscious with complete airway obstruction.

CHOKING IN A RESPONSIVE PERSON

A foreign body lodged in the airway may cause partial or complete airway obstruction. When a foreign body partially blocks the airway, either good or poor air exchange may result.

What to Look For

➤ Partial air exchange
  • Good partial air exchange: victim is still able to cough
  • Poor partial air exchange: victim has a weak, ineffective cough and blue, gray, or ashen skin
➤ Abnormal breathing sounds
  • Snoring: tongue may be blocking airway
  • Crowing: voice box spasm
  • Wheezing: airway swelling or spasm
  • Gurgling: blood, vomit, or other liquid in the airway
➤ Complete blockage (no air exchange)
  • Victim unable to speak, breathe, or cough
  • Victim clutches neck with one or both hands

What to Do

1. Give up to 5 abdominal thrusts (Heimlich maneuver).
   • Stand behind victim.
   • Wrap your arms around victim's waist (do not allow your forearms to touch the ribs).
   • Make a fist with 1 hand and place the thumb side just above victim's navel and well below the lower tip of the breastbone.
   • Grasp your fist with your other hand.
   • Press fist into victim's abdomen, giving 5 quick upward thrusts. Each thrust should be a separate and distinct effort to dislodge the obstructing object. Relieve the abdominal pressure completely between thrusts.

- After every 5 abdominal thrusts, check the victim and your technique.

Note: For the very obese and for women in advanced pregnancy, place your fist on the *lower half of the sternum* instead of the abdomen.

2. Repeat cycles of up to 5 abdominal thrusts until the victim coughs up the object, the victim starts to breathe or coughs forcefully, you are relieved by another trained person, or the victim becomes unresponsive: do a finger sweep and continue using the techniques for the unresponsive adult (below).

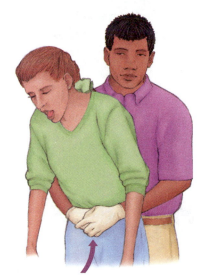

Technique of Heimlich maneuver on responsive victim.

UNRESPONSIVE (UNCONSCIOUS) ADULT WITH FOREIGN BODY AIRWAY OBSTRUCTION (CHOKING)

What to Do

1. Give up to 5 abdominal thrusts.
   - Position victim on a flat, firm surface on his or her back.
   - Straddle victim's thighs.
   - Put heel of one hand against middle of victim's abdomen slightly above navel and well below lower end of breastbone (fingers of hand should point toward victim's head).

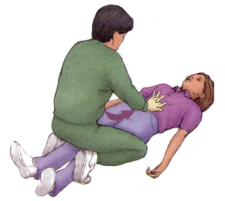

Technique of Heimlich maneuver on unresponsive victim

   - Put other hand directly on top of first hand.
   - Press inward and upward with up to 5 quick abdominal thrusts.

- Each thrust should be a separate and distinct effort to relieve the obstruction. Relieve pressure between thrusts but keep heel of first hand on abdomen.

2. Perform finger sweep of the mouth (use latex gloves, if you have them).
   - Use this maneuver only on unresponsive victim without a gag reflex; otherwise it may cause gagging or vomiting.

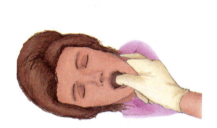
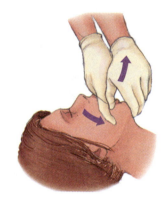

Finger sweep technique

- Use your thumb and fingers to grasp victim's lower jaw and tongue, and lift upward to pull the tongue away from the back of the throat.
- If unable to open the mouth to perform the above, cross the index finger and thumb and push the teeth apart.
- Slide the index finger of your other hand down along the inside of one cheek deeply into mouth, and use a hooking motion across toward the other cheek to dislodge the foreign object.
- If the foreign object comes within reach, grasp and remove it. Do not force the object deeper.

3. If unsuccessful: Repeat cycles of 5 abdominal (or chest) thrusts followed by finger sweep until the object is expelled, you are relieved by another qualified person, or your efforts are unsuccessful after 30 minutes.

CONSCIOUS INFANT WITH FOREIGN BODY AIRWAY OBSTRUCTION (CHOKING)

The infant is responsive but cannot cough, cry, or breathe.

What to Do

1. Give up to 5 back blows.
   - Hold the infant's head and neck with one hand by firmly holding the jaw between your thumb and fingers.
   - Lay the infant facedown over your forearm with the head lower than the chest. Support your forearm on your thigh.
   - Give up to 5 back blows between the infant's shoulder blades with the heel of your hand.

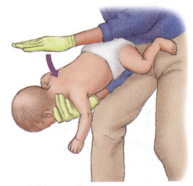

Back blow technique

2. Give up to 5 chest thrusts.
   - Support the back of the infant's head.
   - Sandwich the infant between your hands and forearms and turn the infant over onto his/her back with the head lower than the chest. Small rescuers may need to support the infant on their lap.
   - Locate the proper chest position (same location as for chest compressions in CPR, page 295.)
   - Give up to 5 separate and distinct thrusts with the middle and

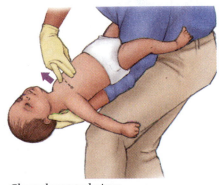

Chest thrust technique

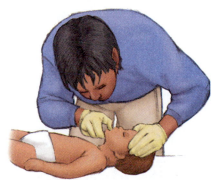

Visual sweeep for foreign object in infant's mouth

ring fingers, similar to CPR chest compressions but at a slower rate.

- Keep fingers in contact with the chest between chest thrusts.

3. Check the mouth for a foreign object.

- Grasp both tongue and jaw between your thumb and fingers and lift.
- If the object is visible, remove it with a finger sweep by sliding the little finger of your other hand alongside the cheek to the base of the tongue using a hooking action.
- Do not do "blind" finger sweeps on an infant or small child in an attempt to remove an unseen object; you may push it deeper.

4. Repeat.

- Give one slow breath (retilt head and try a second slow breath if the first is unsuccessful).
- Give up to 5 back blows.
- Give up to 5 chest thrusts.
- Check the mouth for a foreign object. If you see one, use the finger sweep. Repeat steps until object is expelled or help arrives.

How Can an Untrained Rescuer Help?

An untrained rescuer can go for help, follow instructions to check breathing and pulse, and perform CPR by giving chest compressions while the trained rescuer gives rescue breaths. The untrained rescuer can do 5 chest compressions at the proper rate and depth, stopping while the trained rescuer gives one breath, then starting another cycle with 5 chest compressions.

If the untrained rescuer adequately performs chest compressions, the trained rescuer should allow him or her to continue helping.

APPENDIX B

First Aid Equipment and Supplies

Your wilderness first aid kit deserves careful planning. Consider trip duration, maximum time to medical care, space and weight available for the kit, activities and environmental conditions expected, age and preexisting health conditions of the group members, and the first aid knowledge and experience in the group. You may choose to buy a prepackaged first aid kit or to compile your own.

Carry the items in an easily recognized container such as a red or orange bag. If you anticipate water exposure (heavy rains, river crossings, boating), place individual items in ziplock plastic bags and store the whole kit in a watertight container. Individual members of a group should carry their own kit with a few commonly used items in case they get separated.

The following list contains useful first-aid kit items for a short trip. Modify the list according to the specifics of your group and itinerary. Consult earlier sections of the text for information on additional items.

First Aid Items for a 3- to 4-Day Trip (for 2–3 Persons)

Topical antiseptic towelettes	10
Topical anesthetic cream	1 small tube, or pads
Antibiotic ointment	4 individual packs or 1 small tube
Aloe vera gel	1 small tube
Moleskin/molefoam or Spenco Second Skin™	1 package
Irrigation syringe (20 cc)	1
Bandage strips	10–15 1" strips
Sterile gauze pads	4 @ 2" × 2", 6 @ 4" × 4"
Nonadherent pads	4
Self-adhering roller bandage	1 4" roll
Trauma pad	1 5" × 9" pad
Elastic bandage	1 3" roll
Tape	1 2" roll adhesive or duct tape
Safety pins	3 large
Pain and antiinflammatory medication	10 acetaminophen (Tylenol) tablets, 325 mg
	10 ibuprofen tablets or aspirin, 200 mg
Decongestant	6 tablets
Antihistamine	6 tablets
Hydrocortisone cream	1 small tube, 1%
Sunscreen	1 tube per person, minimum SPF 15
Lip balm (with sunscreen)	1 stick per person
Insect repellent with DEET	1 bottle, plus permanone spray if in tick country
Antacids	8–10 tablets
Antidiarrheal tablets	10 tablets
Povidone-iodine solution	1 oz, 10%
Scissors	1
Tweezers	1
Thermometer	1 (low-reading in cold climate)
Aluminum padded splint (SAM™)	1
Latex gloves	2–4
Pocket mask or microshield	1
Notebook/pencil	1 each

Wound Care (see chapter 4)

First Aid Supplies

	Type/brand/size	Uses, comments	Alternatives/prevention
Blister care supplies	Moleskin, molefoam, Spenco Second Skin™	Treat "hot spots" before blister formation. Pad painful blisters.	Wear a sock liner; break in hiking boots before trip; apply adhesive or duct tape over hot spot.
Irrigation syringe	10 cc or 20 cc syringe with 16–18 gauge flexible catheter tip	High-pressure irrigation of wound to flush dirt and bacteria	Wash with topical antiseptics.
Topical antiseptic	Towelettes with benzalkonium chloride, and/or povidone-iodine solution, 10%, 1 oz	Clean cuts, scrapes, and bites. Iodine solutions can be used for water disinfection (see appendix C).	Soap and water
Topical anesthetic	Ointment, solution, or cleansing pads with lidocaine	Provides some local numbing for cleaning dirt from abrasions and shallow cuts	Ice or cold water
Ophthalmic ointment	Polysporin	Conjunctivitis Corneal abrasions	Do not use nonopthalmic ointments as alternatives.
Antimicrobial ointment	Triple antibiotic ointment Polysporin Neosporin	Provides optimal healing environment, helps prevent skin infections associated with dirty cuts, scrapes and bites. Makes nonstick dressings.	Does not replace meticulous wound cleansing.
Aloe vera	100% gel or various creams with high concentration	Aloe can be used to soothe pain of thermal or sunburn and superficial frostbite.	Antibiotic ointment on burns Caution: some people develop sensitivity/reaction to aloe.

Bandage Material (see chapter 5)

	Type/brand/size	Uses, comments	Alternatives/prevention
Adhesive bandages	Variety of sizes, including strips and "knuckle": Band-Aid™	Cover minor wounds.	Improvise by cutting gauze pad and tape.
Steri-strips	¼" × 4" adhesive strips	Close certain minor, clean wounds.	Can fashion from regular tape; most wounds do not need closure in the wilderness.
Gauze pad dressings	2" × 2" and 4" × 4" sterile pads (individually wrapped packages of 2 pads)	Absorbent wound dressings; carry some sterile and some nonsterile. Nonsterile pads are adequate for most dressings, less expensive and less bulky without packaging.	Cleanest available absorbent, lint-free material
Nonadherent gauze pads	Aquaphor™, Xeroform™, Adaptic™, Telfa™, Spenco Second Skin™, Hydrogel™	Nonadherent pads provide ideal protection for burns, blisters, and scrapes.	Antibiotic ointment on dry gauze or clean cloth creates a nonstick dressing.
Self-adhering gauze	2"–4" wide self-adhering roller gauze: Kerlex™, Kling™	Secure bandages and provide additional padding and barrier; easy to apply.	Clean cloth, elastic wrap
Sterile trauma pads	Highly absorbent pad 5" × 9", 8" × 10"	Dressing for large lacerations, abrasions, open fractures with substantial bleeding or oozing fluid.	Menstrual pads

Bandage Material (see chapter 5) (cont.)

	Type/brand/size	Uses, comments	Alternatives/prevention
Elastic bandage	3–4 inches wide rubberized: ACE Wrap™	Provide compression to reduce swelling and minimal support for joint sprains; pressure dressing; bulky, but often useful.	Cloth strips, roller gauze, athletic tape for sprains
Tape	Porous cloth athletic tape (Zonas™) and/or hypoallergenic "silk" tape, or waterproof tape	Secure bandages and splinting material in place; athletic tape useful for taping sprains.	Tie or pin gauze or elastic wrap; duct tape
Tincture of benzoin	Benzoin liquid 1/2 oz–1 oz or single-use ampules	Adhesive to enhance stickiness of wound closure strips or tape	Athletic tape or duct tape
Safety pins	1"–2" long	Create sling with bandana, cloth, shirt tail or sleeve; hold dressings in place; drain blister; many other uses.	

Nonprescription Medications

	Type/brand/size	Uses, comments	Alternatives/prevention
Anagelsic antipyretics	Acetaminophen (Tylenol™), aspirin, ibuprofen (Advil™, Motrin™), naprosyn (Aleve™)	Treat fever or mild to moderate pain.	
Decongestant tablets	Sudafed™ (decongestant); Actifed™, Dristan™, Contact™, Dimetapp™, others (decongestant/antihistamine)	Relieve nasal and upper respiratory congestion of viral "colds," allergies, and sinus infections, high-altitude runny nose.	Nasal decongestant spray such as Afrin™ or Neosynephrine™; let drip or blow nose
Antihistamine tablets	Diphenhydramine: Benadryl™ (best all-purpose); Chorpheniramine™, Dramamine™, many others	Relieves allergy symptoms of watery eyes, nasal drainage, and hives. Treats itching and rash associated with poison ivy or oak. Causes nausea and motion sickness. Induces sleep.	
Hydrocortisone cream, 1%	Cortaid™, Lanacort™, Cortizone™	Soothes inflammation associated with insect bites, poison ivy, poison oak, and other allergic skin rashes.	Antihistamine tablets or cold compresses; calamine lotion
Antifungal cream	Clotrimazole, mycostatin: Lotrimin™, Micatin™, Nizoral™	Treats athlete's foot and fungal and yeast infections of the groin and vagina. For longer trips, tropics, or susceptible persons.	Attempt prevention by avoiding long periods with wet feet and wet undergarments. Women may get a yeast infection if taking antibiotics.
Sunscreen	Lotion with sun protection factor (SPF) of at least 15, and/or opaque sunblock cream containing zinc oxide or titanium	Prevention of sunburn, windburn. Especially important when traveling on snow or near water.	Minimize sun exposure by wearing a wide-brim hat, lightweight long-sleeved shirt, and pants.

Nonprescription Medications (cont.)

	Type/brand/size	Uses, comments	Alternatives/prevention
Lip balm	Sun protection factor of at least 15; Blistex™ SPF 15 or Chap Stick™ Sunblock 15	Prevents sunburn, chapping of lips. Soothes cold sores.	Opaque sunblock cream containing zinc oxide or titanium
Insect repellent	Those containing DEET; newer preparations longer-acting and contain about 30% DEET; Permanone for ticks	Reduces insect bites. For children, use no more than 10% DEET products. Permanone on clothes repels ticks.	Lightweight long-sleeved shirts, pants tucked into socks, daily tick inspection, mosquito nets
Antacids	Tablets to neutralize acid: Mylanta™, Gelusil™, Tums™	Treat heartburn, acid indigestion	Avoid caffeine, sweets, chocolate, and spicy food; do not eat near bedtime.
Antidiarrheals	Loperamide: Imodium™ capsules, 1 or 2 mg capsules	Decrease diarrhea; victim must also maintain hydration (see appendix D)	Pepto-Bismol™; diet change (see chapter 12); antibiotic for traveler's diarrhea
Oral rehydration salts	WHO formulation: Oralyte™; USA preparations: rehydralyte	When mixed with purified water can help treat dehydration associated with diarrhea, vomiting, and heat exhaustion.	Sports drinks, water with salt and sugar, soup broth (see appendix D)
Oral glucose gel (see chapter 13)	Glucose paste	For victim who may be diabetic. Treats insulin shock. Carry if diabetic person in your group.	Hard candy or sugar if person is conscious

Equipment

	Type/brand/size	Uses, comments	Alternatives/prevention
Water purification system (see appendix C)	Iodine tablets or solutions, filters, chlorine tablets, or solutions	Removal of waterborne germs that can cause intestinal illness; iodine solutions are used for wound cleaning	Boil water. Carry enough water with you from a known "safe" source.
Scissors	Bandage type with blunt ends; paramedic shears; small folding scissors available at sewing stores	Removing victim's clothing; modifying bandage material	Scissors or blade on pocket knife; seam ripper
Tweezers	Fine pointed, splinter forceps: Uncle Bill's Tweezers, Splinter Pickers, Swiss Army knife tweezers	Remove splinters and ticks.	Fingernail, tip of knife, safety pin, needle from sewing kit
Splinting material (see chapter 7)	Malleable foam padded splint such as SAM™ splint, air splints, wire splints, portable traction splints also available	Immobilizing broken bone or severe sprain, emergency neck collar	Many materials for improvisation: boards, branches, ground pad, tent poles, metal stays, adjacent body parts
Thermometer	Usual thermometer ranges from 94°F–105°F. Extended ranges (75°F–105°F) available	For diagnosis of fever; extended range for accurate reading in heatstroke or hypothermia. Carry in a protective case.	Oral temp-dot strips. Determine presence of fever by touch.
Venom extractor kit (see chapter 18)	Sawyer Extractor™	Creates suction over bite site and may remove portion of venom from snake or insect bite. Does not require incision.	Most first aid measures useless, evacuate if signs of envenomation (see chapter 17).

Equipment (cont.)

	Type/brand/size	Uses, comments	Alternatives/prevention
CPR mouth to mask barrier device (see chapter 3)	CPR Microshield, Pocket Mask	Provides "universal precaution" barrier between victim and first aid provider during rescue breathing.	
Latex or vinyl gloves		Protects first aid provider from potentially infected blood and body fluids.	Any barrier like gloves or plastic bags to avoid blood contact with skin; wash skin with soap if exposed.
Notebook		Recording information about injury or illness; sending detailed information to rescuers	Blank page of guide book, first aid book, or paperback book
Writing utensil	Soft, waterproof pencil	Recording information about injury or illness. Pens may leak and do not work in cold.	
Emergency dental kit	Eugenol™ (oil of cloves) for pain relief. Cavit™ temporary filling (small tube, by prescription or from dentist); commercial kits available.	For repair of teeth or relief of pain from cracked tooth, lost fillings or crowns	Candle wax

Prescription Medications

These items should be considered for prolonged remote travel. They require more advanced first aid knowledge, special training, or instructions. The medications require a prescription from a doctor.

	Type/brand/size	Uses, comments	Alternatives/prevention
Asthma kit broncho-dilating inhaler	Nonprescription—epinephrine: Primatene™ Prescription—Ventolin, Proventil, Metaprel	Treatment of asthma attack or wheezing	Nonprescription tablets are available but not as effective.
Antibiotic	Keflex, Bactrim, Erythromycin, Augmentin, Amoxicillin	Treatment of respiratory, skin, and urinary infections. May need more than one kind of antibiotic.	Many different antibiotics with specific indications. Need to discuss with health professional.
Antibiotic for traveler's diarrhea	Cipro, Bactrim, Norfloxacin	For treatment of diarrhea acquired during travel in underdeveloped countries.	Pepto-Bismol, Imodium, or Lomotil; fluid replacement (see appendix D)
Prescription pain medication	Oral narcotics: Tylenol with codeine, Vicodin	Treatment of moderate to severe pain. Helpful for long evacuations over difficult terrain.	Intravenous pain medications administered by licensed provider
Altitude sickness medication (see chapter 15)	Diamox™, Decadron™, Nifedipine™	Prevention and treatment of symptoms of acute mountain sickness. Decadron is for cerebral edema (HACE). Nifedipine is for pulmonary edema.	Slow elevation gain to allow acclimatization; descent
Anaphylaxis kit	Epi-Pen™, Ana-Kit™	Treatment of anaphylactic reaction to bee sting, insect bite, or other severe allergic reaction	Essential if responsible for group or history of previous reaction

	Type/brand/size	Uses, comments	Alternatives/prevention
Traction splint device	DABBS (National Ski Patrol) ski tip and tail adaptor for improvising traction from a ski; Kendrick Traction Device	Traction splinting of long bone fractures for evacuation	Learn to improvise with paddle, ski poles, or nontraction splinting technique
Airway device	Nasal or oral airway	Protection of airway in an unconscious victim; first-aider must know how to use these	Manual techniques (see chapter 3)
Communication equipment	Cellular phone, VHF radio, geographic (GPS) locator	Contact of search and rescue or other authorities	

APPENDIX C
Field Water Disinfection

In the wilderness, the safety of drinking water cannot be assumed. Wilderness travelers usually depend on surface water, which carries a risk of intestinal illness due to bacteria, viruses, and protozoan cysts. Risks vary with geographic location, but while the risk in North America may be small, water treatment is still advised. In countries without good sanitation even tap water should be treated.

Disinfection of water is similar to pasteurization of food products: it makes water bacteriologically safe for drinking. Sterilization, the destruction of all life forms, is not necessary for drinking water, but is preferable for water used in washing wounds.

In North America, the flagellate protozoan *Giardia lamblia* is the most common contaminant in wilderness water, but bacteria and viruses also cause outbreaks of illness. *Cryptosporidium* is common in sewage-contaminated water and is becoming more of a problem in wilderness water.

Methods of Water Disinfection

Heat disinfection depends on the length of exposure and the temperature. Boiling is not essential. Temperatures as low as 140°F (60°C) for 30 minutes are effective, as in pasteurization of food products. Higher temperatures require less time. Disinfection occurs while bringing water to a boil; so, even at high altitude where water boils at a lower temperature, boiled water is safe. To make highly polluted water safe, boil for one minute, or bring to a boil and leave covered for several minutes.

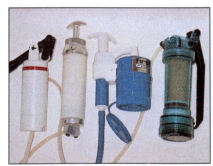

Mechanical filters are appropriate for small-group use in North American wilderness or other areas with high-quality surface water. From left to right: Sweetwater Guardian, Katadyn Pocket Filter, General Ecology First Need, MSR WaterWorks II. (Other products are available.)

TABLE C.1

Average Maximal Filter Pore Size for Removal of Specific Microorganisms	
Microorganism	**Micrometers (μm)**
Giardia, E. histolytica	5
Cryptosporidium	1
Intestinal bacteria	0.4–0.5
Viruses	0.01
Note: Most field filters have a pore size from 0.1–5 μm.	

Filters for wilderness use can remove Giardia, other protozoal cysts, and intestinal bacteria, but they may not remove the much smaller viruses. Some filters incorporate an iodine resin (see Table C.1) to kill viruses and activated charcoal to absorb chemical contaminants.

Clarification techniques remove suspended particulate matter and many microorganisms. They do not disinfect water reliably but may improve clarity and taste and improve the efficacy of filtration or halogenation.

Sedimentation separates large particles by gravity. Allow water to stand in a container for at least one hour, then pour off the clear portion.

Charcoal filters (purifiers) alone are not adequate for disinfection. They improve taste and appearance of water by absorbing chemicals but do not absorb all microorganisms.

Coagulation/flocculation removes smaller suspended particles that will not settle with gravity. The technique works best on "cloudy" water, such as brown or green water that is loaded with organic material. Add 1/8 to 1/4 teaspoon alum (aluminum sulfate) per gallon of water and mix thoroughly. Then stir or gently agitate occasionally for 5 minutes and allow to settle; colloidal particles flocculate (clump together) and layer out. The clear water can be decanted, filtered, or poured through a cloth or coffee filter. The majority of microorganisms will settle with the floc, but for safety use a second disinfection step. Alum can be obtained at chemical supply stores or some grocery stores (as pickling powder).If alum is not available, powdered lime or the fine white ash from a campfire can be used.

Halogens (chlorine and iodine) are effective disinfectants for viruses, bacteria, and protozoan cysts (except Cryptosporidium). Both are available in tablet or liquid form. Iodine also comes in crystalline and resin form. In equivalent concentrations, iodine has some advantages over chlorine for field use (see Table C.2).

The effectiveness of a halogen depends on its concentration and the length of time it is left in the water (contact time). Weaker concen-

Coagulation-flocculation

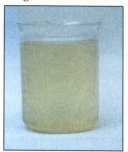 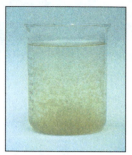 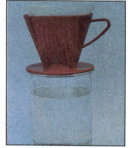

| Cloudy water from a pond laden with suspended organic particles (colloids) that will not settle out. | After adding about 1/8 tsp of alum (aluminum sulfate) and stirring, clumps of floc form. | After the floc has settled, pour through a fine-weave cloth or coffee filter to obtain clear water. The poor taste, smell, and color have been removed. This water should be treated or pumped through a water filter to remove remaining microorganisms. |

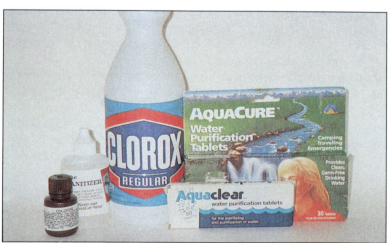

Sources of chlorine for water treatment
From left to right: Sanitizer method of superchlorination-dechlorination; household bleach (5% sodium hypochlorite); Aquaclear tablets; AquaCure tablets for flocculation and chlorination.

trations or colder water require longer contact times. If high doses are used, the taste becomes unpleasant. Smaller doses are effective in clear water with prolonged contact time.

Because iodine and chlorine react with organic impurities to form a relatively inactive compound, their doses must be increased in grossly contaminated or cloudy water. Inorganic particulate matter, like sand and clay, does not

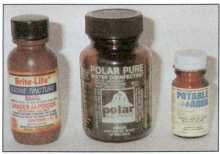

Sources of iodine for water treatment
From left to right: 2% tincture of iodine;
Polar Pure iodine crystals in water (saturated solution of iodine); Potable Aqua tablets.

react with halogens but can be removed by straining, filtering, or sedimentation to improve taste. It is best to clarify cloudy water before treatment with halogens.

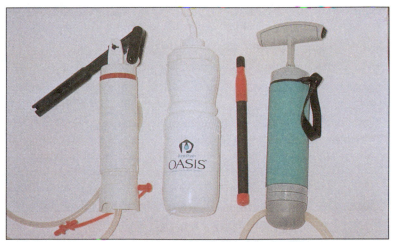

Examples of filters incorporating iodine resin for water treatment (other products are available). These filters are appropriate for domestic wilderness water or water with risk of high contamination from human waste, such as water in undeveloped countries. From left to right: SweetWater Guardian with Viral Guard attachment; Water Technology Corporation (WTC) Oasis; Straw with resin and filtration (not recommended except for survival situations); PUR Explorer.

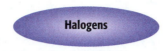

TABLE C.2

Advantages	Disadvantages
Chlorine	
Inexpensive	Moisture, heat, and air affect potency
Available in multiple forms	Will stain or bleach if spilled on clothes
Allows flexibility in dosing	Requires knowledge to use correctly
Taste can be neutralized	Adds taste to water
Iodine	
Taste is better tolerated than chlorine	Active in body, toxic in high doses
Less reactive with water contaminants	Not recommended for:
Wider choice of preparations available	• unstable thyroid disease
Preparations are more stable	• known iodine allergy
	• longer than 1–3 weeks in pregnant women: use longer than a few months in others

The taste of halogens in water may be improved by several means:

- Decrease the amount of halogen while increasing the contact time.
- Add flavored drink mix *after* adequate contact time.
- Pass the water through a charcoal filter *after* adequate contact time.
- Use techniques that do not leave residual halogen, such as heat or filters.
- Neutralize the taste of iodine or chlorine by adding a pinch of ascorbic acid (vitamin C) or using hydrogen peroxide in combination with calcium hypochlorite (see Table C.3). All of these techniques chemically change iodine to iodide or chlorine to chloride.

Special Techniques for Water Disinfection
IODINE RESINS (PENTAPURE AND TRIOCIDE)

The resin releases iodine "on demand," on contact with microorganisms. The exact mechanism of iodine transfer to organisms is not known. Many filters include a charcoal resin to remove any iodine dissolved in the water after passing through the iodine resin. Some devices incorporate a microfilter to remove cysts that are more resistant to iodine. Because of the iodination, these filters destroy viruses in water.

TABLE C.3

Disinfection Techniques
and Halogen Doses

Iodination Techniques	Amount for 4 ppm	Amount for 8 ppm
All doses added to 1 quart water Iodine tabs Tetraglycine hydroperiodide EDWGT (emergency drinking water germicidal tablet) Potable Aqua Globaline	1 tab in 2 qts	1 tab in 1 qt
2% iodine solution (tincture)*	0.2 ml 5 drops	0.4 ml 10 drops
Saturated iodine crystals in water; can measure with bottlecap (Commercial name: Polar Pure)	13 ml	26 ml

Chlorination Techniques	Amount for 5 ppm	Amount for 10 ppm
Halazone (monodichloraminobenzoic acid) Aquaclear (sodium dichloroisocyanurate) Household bleach 5%* sodium hypochlorite *Measure with dropper (1 drop = 0.05 ml) or small syringe	2 tabs 1 tab/2 qts 0.1 ml 2 drops	4 tabs 1 tab/1 qt 0.2 ml 4 drops

In cloudy or polluted water, some contact time (15 to 30 minutes) should be allowed before drinking. Commercial products are made by Water Technologies Corporation, Recovery Engineering (Pur filters), and SweetWater (Viral Guard).

SATURATED IODINE CRYSTALS

This is the most stable iodine solution: four grams of iodine crystals in a 2-oz glass bottle filled with water. Decant iodine-saturated water (leaving undissolved crystals at the bottom of the bottle) into the drinking water. Refill the iodine bottle with water to make new batches of disinfection solution. The bottle may be refilled many times before all crystals have dissolved. The solution will become saturated with iodine within 20 minutes in warm water, but wait 1 hour if using very cold

TABLE C.4

Contact Time before Use between Agent and Water at Various Water Temperatures

Concentration of Halogen	40°F (5°C)	60°F (15°C)	85°F (30°C)
2 ppm	240 min.	180 min.	60 min.
4 ppm	180 min.	60 min.	45 min.
8 ppm	60 min.	30 min.	15 min.

Notes: Very cold water requires prolonged contact time with iodine or chlorine to kill *Giardia* cysts. These contact times in cold water have been extended from the usual recommendations to account for this and for the uncertainty of residual concentration. In cloudy water that will not settle out by sedimentation, the dose of halogen should be at least 8 ppm to account for greater halogen demand from organic material. Even better, use coagulation-flocculation to clarify the water first, then the usual doses of halogen.

water. The dose of saturated iodine solution is calculated for room temperature. If the crystal bottle is very cold, warm by putting it in your pocket or increase the dose by 30%.

Iodine crystals can also be placed in ethyl alcohol, creating a more concentrated solution. The dose is 0.1 ml (2 drops) for 4 ppm and 0.2 ml (4 drops) for 8 ppm.

IODINE TABLETS

These are the simplest to use, requiring no measurement. Since they are concentrated, 1 tablet can be added to 2 quarts of water, with prolongation of the contact time. Potable Aqua iodine tablets now come with "neutralizing" tablets—ascorbic acid—which can be added after the contact time to remove color and taste. This does not remove iodine but converts it to iodide, which still has effects within the body. Tablets decompose over time. Once a bottle has been opened the tablets will remain effective for 12 months.

CHLORINATION/DECHLORINATION

This technique uses very high concentrations of chlorine for disinfection, then dechlorinates with peroxide, which forms soluble calcium chloride, a tasteless and odorless compound. Excess peroxide bubbles off as oxygen. The kit consists of chlorine crystals (calcium hypochlorite) and 30% hydrogen peroxide in separate small nalgene bottles.

This is a very good technique for highly polluted or cloudy waters, for disinfecting large volumes, and for storing water on boats. (Commercially available as The Sanitizer and Sierra Water Purifier.)

Note: Thirty percent hydrogen peroxide is corrosive and burns skin.

CHLORINATION/FLOCCULATION

Tablets contain a flocculating agent and chlorine compound to clarify water and provide residual chlorine concentration. The remaining sediment is removed by pouring through a simple cloth, paper, or other filter. This technique is best for cloudy water; in clear water the flocculating agent leaves some unwanted sediment. Flocculation has the advantage of removing most cysts that are less susceptible to chlorine. The residual chlorine concentration is variable and may be fairly strong, up to 10 mg per liter.

Choice of Technique

The best technique depends on personal preference and intended use. Use of heat may be limited by fuel supplies. For a large group, halogenation or high-capacity filters are convenient. As water quality deteriorates, two-stage techniques become more important; for example, clarification by flocculation or filtration, followed by halogenation.

Filtration is not a reliable method for removing viruses. Halogens do not kill *Cryptosporidium*, a protozoal organism. Although viral and *Cryptosporidium* contamination is currently a low risk in North American alpine surface water, high levels of contamination should be assumed in lowland rivers with towns upstream and in undeveloped countries.

TABLE C.5

Effectiveness of Disinfection Methods for Microorganisms

	Heat	Filters	Halogens
Bacteria	yes	yes	yes
Viruses	yes	no	yes
Protozoa	yes	yes	
Giardia, ameba			yes
Cryptosporidium			no

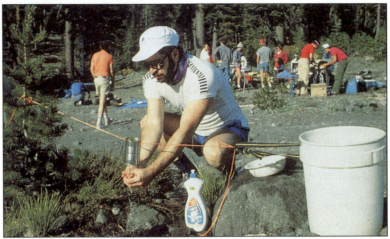

Camp hygiene: hand washing

Thus, only two methods are effective against all waterborne enteric pathogens: heat or a combination of filtration and halogens (or iodine resin/microfiltration units). These techniques must be used for high risk areas noted above. For North American "pristine" wilderness water, any single technique is probably reasonable.

Camp Hygiene

Proper hygiene prevents contamination of groundwater and limits the spread of illness among group members.

WASTE DISPOSAL IN AREAS WITHOUT TOILETS OR GROUP LATRINES

- Dig a hole 8" to 10" deep to bury waste.
- Dig at least 100 feet from surface water, and do not dig in natural drainages where the first rain could wash waste into the water source.
- Burn or bury toilet paper with waste and stamp down or cover with a rock.
- For large groups or high-use areas, dig a common trench latrine. After each use, sprinkle a little dirt on the waste.
- Carry a small plastic spade or collapsible shovel or improvise with a stick or flat spade-shaped rock.

PERSONAL HYGIENE

Always wash hands after going to the bathroom and before preparing food. Place a bucket of water, dipper, and soap along the path to the latrine or next to the cooking area.

GROUP HYGIENE

- Use utensils rather than hands to serve food.

- When washing dishes, add bleach to the final rinse water. Carry a few ounces of liquid or powder bleach (1 to 2 oz should suffice for a small group for 1 week). Add enough to create a strong smell of chlorine. Allow dishes to air dry.

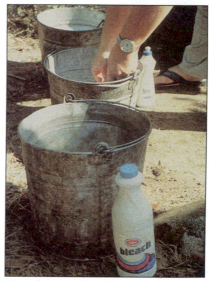

Camp hygiene: bleach in rinse water

APPENDIX D
Fluid and Electrolyte Replacement

Oral rehydration/electrolyte solutions (ORS) are useful in four circumstances when fluids and electrolytes are lost in significant amounts: severe diarrhea and/or vomiting; treatment of mild to moderate heat illness; heavy, prolonged exercise with high-volume sweat loss; and injury with significant blood loss or fluid loss from burns.

Replacement of Intestinal Fluid Losses

Diarrhea (e.g., traveler's diarrhea) is the main reason for using oral electrolyte solutions. Most intestinal infections resolve by themselves, but they cause the loss of fluid and electrolytes and can result in dehydration. Even during severe diarrhea, the gut can absorb water and electrolytes when mixed with glucose.

The World Health Organization has developed electrolyte salts specifically for diarrheal illness that contain sodium, potassium, chloride, bicarbonate or trisodium citrate, and glucose; these should be mixed with 1 quart of disinfected water. Packets of these oral rehydration salts are distributed throughout the world by WHO and UNICEF, commonly under the name of Oralyte. In the United States, the WHO salts and rice-based solutions are hard to find. More expensive premixed solutions are available but impractical for wilderness or foreign travel.

Recipe for Making ORS Powder	
Add to 1 liter of disinfected water:	
potassium chloride (KCl)	1.5 gm
baking soda	2.5 gm
salt (NaCl)	3.5 gm
glucose	20.0 gm

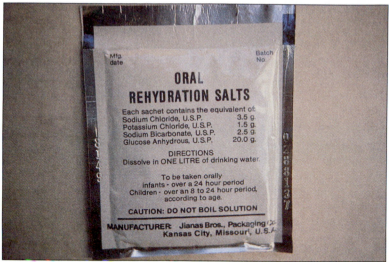

Oral rehydration salts

Cereal-based ORS contains complex carbohydrate molecules from rice or grains that are digested as simple glucose. Sports drinks and other "clear liquids" contain too little sodium and potassium and too much glucose for treating diarrhea-induced dehydration, but they may be better than plain water (see Table D.2).

If premeasured salts are not available, a substitute recommended by the Centers for Disease Control consists of alternating drinks of the following two fluids:

Glass 1:   8 oz fruit juice (apple, orange, lemonade, etc.)
1/2 tsp honey or corn syrup
1 pinch salt
Glass 2:   8 oz water (boiled or treated)
1/4 tsp baking soda

Some ingredients may not be available in remote locations.

Plain salt-and-sugar solutions, similar to those used for heat/exercise replacement, can be used for mild dehydration but are not adequate for serious dehydration or replacing continuing high losses. For mild dehydration, partial maintenance, supplementation, or where nothing else is available, rice water, fruit juice, coconut milk, diluted cola drinks, or soup broth may suffice.

GUIDELINES FOR FLUID REPLACEMENT

Estimated fluid deficit should be replaced in about 4 hours. For mild dehydration, an adult should drink 8 ounces of ORS every 30 minutes for the first 4 to 6 hours. Children should drink 6 to 8 oz of ORS per hour and as much water as they want. Give infants under 3 months a 4-oz dose each hour, with every third dose replaced by plain water. To prevent vomiting, the person should drink frequent small amounts slowly. Determine maintenance requirements by estimating or measuring stool losses plus normal maintenance requirements. Since this is not often possible in the field, give at least 1 teaspoon (5 ml) per pound of body weight after each diarrheal stool.

Try to continue feeding. Basic grains and starches (the nutritional mainstay in most parts of the world) do not increase or prolong fluid losses. Rice-based ORS may reduce the illness associated with diarrhea. Most staple foods, such as cereals, bananas, lentils, potatoes, fruits, yogurt, and other cooked vegetables are well tolerated and can be continued during diarrhea. Avoid caffeine, alcohol, foods with high sugar concentrations, and fried or fatty foods. Intolerance to dairy products (gas, bloating, and persistent diarrhea) may follow an intestinal illness. Infants may continue breastfeeding. Dilute lactose formula 50% with water and observe for lactose intolerance.

FLUID REPLACEMENT DURING EXERCISE

Sweat losses of 1 qt per hour are common during moderate exercise in a hot, humid environment or heavy exertion in a temperate environment. Dehydration increases the risk of heat illness.

In high-altitude mountaineering, scarcity of surface water, difficulty adjusting clothing to changing weather or levels of exertion, and respiratory fluid losses from hyperventilation in dry cold air commonly create fluid needs of 7 to 8 qt per day. Dehydration at high altitude increases the likelihood of altitude sickness, hypothermia, frostbite, and venous thrombosis.

During sustained hard exercise, especially in a hot environment, a person needs at least 16 oz (1 pint) before exercising and 8 oz every 20 minutes while exercising. The person should drink at every opportunity and gauge hydration by the volume and color of urine. Use only clean water for fluid replacement (see water disinfection, appendix C).

Sweat contains sodium, chloride, and small amounts of potassium. In the wilderness, salt and other electrolyte needs are best replaced by regular meals and snacks, with fluid loss replaced with plain water. In addition, food will provide more calories than electrolyte solutions and enhance fluid intake. Unfortunately, many hikers favor snack foods that are high in carbohydrates and fats (e.g., candy) but low in sodium. Some individuals, noting the swelling present in their hands and feet associated with heat or altitude exposure, mistakenly attempt to restrict their sodium intake.

Electrolyte supplements are advised in endurance events or sustained work/exercise longer than 6 hours; or for a shorter period, in a very hot environment with high sweat losses. Severe hyponatremia (low salt content in the body) that causes confusion and even seizures can occur in endurance athletes and recreational hikers in hot climates.

During exercise, a solution containing 2% to 6% glucose and 30 mEq/L sodium is palatable. Excessive sodium can cause nausea, and salt tablets swallowed whole cause gastric irritation and vomiting. So, dissolve one or two tablets in a liter of water. Too much sugar may delay stomach emptying and cause diarrhea. Commercial sports drinks are available in powder form but simple substitutes can be made at home (see Table D.1).

TREATMENT OF MILD HEAT ILLNESS

Oral electrolyte solutions are excellent for treating mild or moderate heat illness, such as heat syncope, heat cramps, and heat exhaustion. The victim must rest in the shade and sip 1 to 2 quarts of fluids similar to exercise replacement fluids. Oral fluids cannot be used for treating heatstroke with altered consciousness and inability to swallow.

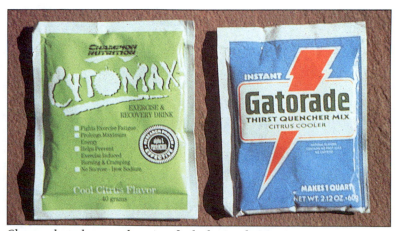

Glucose-electrolyte powder mixes for hydration during exercise

TABLE D.1

Home Sports Solution for Rehydration

Add to 1 Quart of Water	Resulting Concentration
3–4 tsp sugar	1%–2% solution, 50KCal
1/2 tsp table salt	30 mEq/L

The teaspoon measurement is quite variable (3.5–5.0 grams/tsp), but the resulting concentration is fine in these solutions.

Note: Milliequivalents (mEq) is a measure of substances related to both weight and electrical charge; 1.0 liter (L) = 1.05 quarts.

TABLE D.2

Concentrations of Electrolytes in Common Fluids

	Sodium mEq/L	Potassium mEq/L	Bicarbonate mEq/L	Glucose grams/liter
Blood	140	4.5	25	
Diarrhea	50–140	15–25	20–45	
Sweat	30–60	3–5		
Sports drink	10–25	3–5		60–70 (6%–7%)
WHO ORS	90	20	30	20 (2%)
U.S. ORS	45–75	20–25	30	20–25
Soft drinks	2–5	0		110
Orange juice	0–5	58		118

Note: Milliequivalents (mEq) is a measure of substances related to both weight and electrical charge; 1.0 liter (L) = 1.05 quarts.

FLUID AND ELECTROLYTE REPLACEMENT FOR BLOOD LOSS

The fluid lost with serious, continued bleeding cannot be replaced by mouth. But if sudden blood loss has occurred and subsequently stopped (e.g., a wound, nosebleed, or uterine bleeding), oral fluid replacement can help restore blood volume but will not replace lost blood cells. Extensive skin burns lose large volumes of fluid. Give fluids with salt, similar to diarrheal replacement fluids, until intravenous fluids are available.

APPENDIX E

Improving the Odds of Survival

During any wilderness outing, you could be forced to spend an unexpected night out because of an unfamiliar trail, injury, illness, or sudden weather change. Good planning can turn a crisis into an adventure. The following items may improve the odds of survival, which depends as much on determination, skill, and judgment as on equipment.

Clothing

To prevent serious heat loss, always take the minimum amount of extra clothing for comfort in a bad storm.

First Layer   Light to midweight synthetic long underwear (e.g., polypropylene, Thermostat, or Capilene) provide warmth and absorb or wick moisture from skin. All materials lose insulating properties when wet, but cotton loses more than most.

Insulating Layers   Pile or fleece jackets and vests, wool shirts and sweaters, and wool or pile pants

Wind/Rain Layers   Windproof, waterproof, and breathable (e.g., Gore-Tex) for both upper and lower body. Uncoated nylon is sufficient only for wind and light precipitation.

Hat   Wool, pile, or waterproof material that covers the ears. A balaclava or ski hat and neck gaiter provide more warmth than a simple hat and protect the face from frostbite.

Mittens/Gloves   Mittens are warmer than gloves. Wear a synthetic liner as well as a wind/waterproof outer shell. Wool socks make a good substitute for mittens.

Footwear   Wear a polypropylene liner under wool or fleece socks. Boots should be ankle high, have a good traction sole, and be water repellent. Plastic bags between sock layers provide a vapor barrier that increases warmth but may also increase moisture.

Shelter

To conserve heat beyond the insulation provided by clothes, make a shelter by finding a natural cave or windbreak, digging a snow cave or snow trench, or building a quinzhee hut in the snow. Carry a collapsible shovel to build snow shelters and for avalanche rescue. An effective shelter can be rigged up with rope, cord or wire, and a tarp, rainfly, or even a garbage bag. A tent is ideal but not always available. Bivvy sacs provide a lot of warmth for their size and weight; two large garbage bags can function as a light bivvy sac or rain suit. Putting the feet into a backpack offers some protection.

> **Survival adage: A person can survive 3 minutes without oxygen, 3 hours in severe weather without shelter, 3 days without water, 3 weeks without food.**

Water and Food

Water   To melt snow you need a metal container, stove (and fuel if above the timberline), or campfire. A piece of aluminum foil, a black plastic garbage bag, or a space blanket can gather enough sunlight to melt snow and ice. A candle can be used for cooking and melting snow, and for warmth in a snow cave. Carry a wide-mouth canteen filled with water. If possible, disinfect drinking water (see appendix C), but maintaining hydration takes precedence over disinfecting water.

Emergency Food Supply   Always carry emergency food rations. Take food that can be eaten without cooking to minimize preparation time and effort; but a cup of hot soup can do wonders for the psyche. Hard candy, energy bars, jerky, and bouillon cubes are compact and lightweight. Carry a pot and metal cup for cooking. Knowledge of edible native food sources will help.

Heat

Know how to light a fire with minimal resources.

Stove and Fuel   These provide the best source of heat for glacier or desert travel,where wood is scarce. In a forest, firestarters and a folding saw maybe useful.

Matches in Waterproof Container   These work better than a lighter, which may not vaporize in the cold. Carry several sets in different waterproof containers.

Magnesium Firestarters   An alternative to matches, these can be scraped with a steel file or knifeblade, producing sparks to ignite fine-grade steel wool, lint, moss, etc.

Candle   Provides light and enough heat to melt snow or warm a drink.

Ground Insulation   To decrease conductive heat loss, do not sit or lie directly on cold ground. Sit on an ensolite pad (at least 18" square) or Therm-A-Rest pad, your backpack, or pine boughs to insulate from the ground.

Toilet Paper   Can be used as a firestarter; not necessary to survive, but helps for comfort.

Light

Flashlight   Carry fresh batteries and a spare bulb.

Headlamp   Frees your hands.

Candle   Provides minimal light by itself but can be used in a lantern for additional range.

Emergency lightsticks such as the Cyalume Lightstick can provide several hours of dim light. They have a limited shelf-life and often don't work well in the cold.

Route Finding and Navigation

Map and Compass   Carry a topographical map of the area. Know how to read it and how to use a compass for finding your way and checking your location.

Altimeter   Useful in positioning yourself on a topographical map based on known elevation.

Global Positioning System (GPS)   For expeditions and offtrack remote vehicle travel; an advanced navigational tool that uses satellites to pinpoint your location on a longitude/latitude scale. Very accurate; can show your route and indicate direction of travel to return to a previous location.

Travel Aids

Snow and Ice Aids   Cross-country skis (wax and skins), snowshoes, crampons, ice axe, ropes

Rescue Equipment   Rope, harnesses, pulleys, carabiniers, ascenders

Protection Devices   For rock, snow, or ice, depending on the type of travel

Avalanche Beacons and Rescue Equipment   Shovel and probe poles (special ski poles) are important tools for backcountry skiers and hikers traveling on unstable or unknown snowpack.

Surveyor's tape to mark route if going for help, to mark location for air search, and to use as a windsock for helicopter rescue.

Tools and Repair Kit

Multifunction Knife   Swiss Army Knife™ or Leatherman tool™, which provides pliers.

Duct Tape   Can be used to fix just about anything. Wrap a supply around a ski pole, water bottle, or pencil.

Snare, Baling, or Picture Hanging Wire   For tying or fastening and for backpack repairs

Carpet Thread and Heavy-Duty Needle

Safety Pins   Many uses, large sizes preferred

Braided Nylon Cord (50 ft)   Many uses

First Aid Supplies   For treating illness or injury (see appendix B).

Communication Equipment   For contacting others for help or to notify them that all is well.

Whistle (plastic)   Much more effective and efficient than shouting to alert others of trouble; the human voice carries only short distances in the outdoors and gives out quickly. Each member should carry a whistle around his or her neck. Especially useful for children.

Signal Mirror   To signal overhead aircraft or search parties

Flares   Useful for signaling, but heavy

Cellular Phone Compact and lightweight means of calling for help or notifying potential rescuers of your condition. Works only where cellular phone networks are available.

VHF Radio In remote areas can provide radio link with telephone network or contact with authorities monitoring emergency bands. Check with local authorities regarding restricted frequencies.

Vehicle Survival Gear

Bottled water	Sleeping bag or	Fire extinguisher
Flares	blankets	Windshield scraper
Tools	Jumper cables	Road maps
Short hose	Flashlight	Matches and cook pot
(to siphon gas)	Chains	First aid kit
Nonperishable food	Tow cable	Shovel and sand

Ground Signals for Aircraft

Search and rescue is commonly done by aircraft. Ground symbols can be used to signal aircraft so that the victims can remain in a shelter or proceed to find water or safer ground. Make markings in an open area, visible from above. Make designs 8 to 10 feet tall and use items that contrast with the background. Three repetitive symbols indicates distress. An arrow indicates that you are traveling in that direction. A large **X** means you are near that location and unable to proceed.

Additional Photo and Illustration Credits

332

Index

Quick Emergency Index

350